D1458495

THE NATURAL HOME PHYSICIAN

By the same author:
ABOUT DANDELIONS
BIOCHEMIC PRESCRIBER
BIOCHEMISTRY UP-TO-DATE
BUILDING A HEALTHY HEART
HEALTH FROM EARTH, AIR AND WATER
HEALTH FROM THE KITCHEN
KELP: THE HEALTH GIVER
LADY BE BEAUTIFUL
THE GROUP REMEDY PRESCRIBER
TRANQUILLIZATION WITH HARMLESS HERBS

THE NATURAL
HOME PHYSICIAN

by

ERIC F. W. POWELL, Ph.D., N.D.

HEALTH SCIENCE PRESS
1 Church Path, Saffron Walden, Essex,
England

First published 1962
Second Edition, revised, enlarged and reset,
1975
Reprinted 1981

© ERIC F. W. POWELL 1975

*All rights reserved. No part of this publication may be
reproduced or tramsmitted in any form or by any means,
electronic or mechanical, including photocopy, recording, or any
information storage and retrieval system, without permission in
writing from the publisher.*

ISBN 0 85032 092 5

Printed in England by
Hillman Printers Ltd., Frome, Somerset

FOREWORD

In this modern scientific age we tend to pin our faith to the difficult and complex. Unless a medicinal formula contains most of the letters in the alphabet some doubt exists as to its value; while the old remedies, the value of which has been proved by the acid test of time, are neglected and cast aside as being 'far too simple'. But what are the facts?

Many modern drugs are dangerous. They produce 'side effects' which can, in some instances, be more serious than the diseases for which they are prescribed. Not so very long ago aspirin was hailed as a wonder drug, and was expected to cure all sorts of things and conditions associated with pain. But all that aspirin does is to stun the nerves and the brain so that pain does not register. It does not cure the basic cause of pain; although it so happens that sometimes the forced rest of the numbed mind helps the organism to eliminate the cause. But forced rest by drugs, and, to use the modern term, 'tranquilization', can do much harm if persisted with. Only by cause removal can real health be established.

Is it not reasonable to suppose that the Intelligence which, operating through the ages to form the human organism, also gave to it the necessary power to repair and heal itself? What heals a cut finger? The ointment that is applied? No! The repair is done by and through the blood. It is exactly the same with the many diseases to which the flesh is heir: disease is brought about by wrong thinking and faulty living. The healing power in the blood can restore most people to good health if it is supplied with the *natural* elements required for the work of repair. When we consider the quantities of poisoned, chemicalised food eaten day after day it is a wonder that the blood of the average civilised (?)

person can heal anything! 'The life is in the blood' is an
ancient saying, and a true one. Actually, sane feeding and
living to principle will cure anything that is curable. It has
been said that there are no incurable diseases, but there are
incurable people.

The organism is so constructed that it can only utilise to
the best effect substances supplied by nature through the
medium of plant and animal life. Indeed, there is enough
evidence to show that the ideal source of life and vitality is
the vegetable kingdom; but this is not intended to be an
argument for or against the employment of animal food —
that is not the writer's object in these pages. What is to be
stressed is that the body is not designed to deal with crude
mineral matter, or combinations of toxic and mineral
substances no matter what impressive name such a mixture
may have. Of course minerals affect the body. Homoeopathy
proves that. Orthodox medicine also proves it; but such
effects are pathological. In many instances the major effect
of a modern drug is to stimulate the system to get rid of it,
and this stirring-up process may result in the system throwing
off the disease as well, but at the expense of the sufferer's
vitality. Or, the drug may so stun the brain and nerves that
the sufferer thinks he is well, only to discover later on that he
has another disease.

Of course poisonous drugs kill bacteria; but what are
bacteria? Where we have filth the flies gather, and when there
are morbid accumulations within the system we find germs;
for, like all scavengers, germs breed and feed on noxious
substances. It sometimes happens that by killing the germs
some symptoms may disappear — for a time. But has the
cause, the reason why the germs found lodgement in the
body, been removed? The answer is a positive NO! Pure
blood is the finest germicide in the world, and if we get the
blood pure, balanced and organised, germs, other than those
forms of bacteria essential to the life processes, cannot exist in
it. A campaign of germ slaughter will not win the battle
against disease, and one of the world's greatest physicians has
said that doctors pay too much attention to the germ, and not
enough to the host of the germ.

More and more scientists are coming to this conclusion,
and getting back to nature is not quite the quackery that it

was formerly labelled. Scientists have now discovered that certain remedial herbs used by herbalists for hundreds of years have virtues greater than those possessed by the much publicized modern drugs. Hypericum (St. John's Wort) and Symphytum (Comfrey) being examples. But what will these scientists do? They will isolate some 'principle' in the plants which the great chemical firms will eagerly seize upon, give this substance a very learned name, and hail it as a new medical discovery. Fortunes will be made out of it. But it will prove, finally, to be far less effective than was thought. Why? Because nature never intended a principle to be isolated from its organic setting in the plant, where it acts in harmony with substances associated with it. Man has always tried to improve on nature, but when it comes to the unnatural substitution of nature's remedies by a creation of the human brain for the purpose of healing a disorganised human organism, man will never be completely successful. Man's creations are amazing. Only a fool would say otherwise; although these inventions do not always lead to happiness — much the reverse. But man cannot create life, and to maintain life in what nature has created we must take living substances from nature; for nature is the mother who feeds us and we must be nourished from her breasts alone.

The remedies and treatments suggested in this book are not intended to replace the services of the trained healer. In fact it is important that when symptoms are serious professional services should always be obtained, and as quickly as possible. Yet it is astonishing what the average intelligent person can do at home to prevent disease, and an ounce of prevention is worth a ton of cure.

We will even go as far as to say that quite often, when medical science has failed, the suggestions herein may perform what was considered to be impossible; for when we work with nature we have on our side a creative and not a destructive intelligence. The life force in the organism will eagerly take up the healing elements from natural sources and utilise them in no uncertain manner.

The remedies given will not suppress; they will not drive into the organism morbid matter which nature is trying to eliminate. It must be remembered that every acute disease is an effort of the body to throw off a toxic state, and that repeated suppression with poisons can only result in chronic illness, sooner or later. Even the common cold, for which medical science is still trying to find a cure, is a sort of systematic spring-cleaning process. There are some very potent herbal treatments for colds, although the real cure is to cleanse the system and build up the vitality so that the reason for this self-cleansing effort becomes unnecessary. Likewise, a fever is also a burning-up process. It should not be suppressed, but merely controlled with remedies which are non-suppressive, and the system strengthened to throw off the basic causes.

Chronic disease is the result of the continued suppression of acute conditions, of wrong thinking and faulty living. True, a weak constitution can be handed down from one's parents; all the more reason why such a constitution should be built up in a natural manner. Nature will never let anybody down if the game of life is played according to the rules. To put it in a nutshell: when the cause is removed, the effect (the disease) ceases.

Man is not just mind and body; he has a spiritual nature as well. Since man is a triune being he cannot experience true health unless he is adjusted on all three planes of his being. When mind, body or spiritual nature are out of harmony with God and with nature (with TRUTH) man is dis-eased.

Pain is nature's warning that something is wrong. To kill the pain with a drug smothers the warning. There are plenty of natural pain-killers without having to resort to poisons, and natural remedies which remove pain do so by helping to eliminate the cause. Without pain and discomfort we should never know what was wrong in the body. The thing is to heed the warning and put matters right. When medicine fails we admit that surgery comes into its own, and the modern surgeon is a highly skilled fellow who accomplishes miracles with a knife. Often operations are necessary, but so often this necessity is due to erroneous medication. How often we hear that the operation was successful, but the patient died. The teachings in this book will do much to make operations unnecessary.

Famous old cures have been dug out of the past and presented in a manner that all can understand. An effort has been made to discard all the 'old wives' tales', stupid superstitions and anything that savours of 'magic'. Recipes have been tried and tested, and everything recommended is utterly harmless. Old fashioned remedies and methods employed by native peoples have been carefully investigated before inclusion, and the writer himself has had over forty years professional experience to help him. To the sceptical we say: 'Fools deride; philosophers investigate'.

Not many people have the time or the inclination to read a book with long, drawn-out arguments on practical matters that need take only a paragraph or two; and this certainly applies to the busy housewife. It is for her that this effort has been made in particular. Hence, there is but little theorising; but, what we may term, a tabloid presentation of facts and information of intense practical value. To simplify matters the subjects have been arranged in the form of an A-B-C. All the reader has to do is to look up the information desired under the alphabetical heading.

The usefulness of this book will be enhanced by the reader learning as much as possible about each complaint and remedy and it will be observed that, in many instances, more than one remedy is mentioned under the complaint being discussed and it is recommended that, where the other remedies are included under their own headings, the reader should study the information given about each medicine. For instance, under Abscess mention is made of Slippery Elm and Marshmallow so it is advisable to read what is said about these two remedies under their own headings. The same advice applies to remedies; where one or more ailments are mentioned look for each under its own heading. For instance, under Agrimony, Indigestion is dealt with so the information given under the heading of this complaint should be studied.

Herbal remedies with an initial capital letter are dealt with in the appropriate place but this does not apply to Homoeopathic and Biochemic medicines.

These pages are packed with sound, helpful advice and wisdom gleaned from a variety of sources, old and new. It is the author's hope that the information given will enable readers to enjoy healthier and happier lives.

In all matters be governed by reason and sound judgement, and not by faddy ideas.

'Everyone who will look through the history of medical opinion, as regards public health, during the last fifty years, and the amount of money spent in obedience to medical opinion, will find as great a crop of errors, and as large an expenditure of public money which subsequent knowledge has shown to be ill-spent, as anything connected with the Army and Navy. It is regrettable, but it is inevitable. As long as the House of Commons is not entirely composed of men possessing the wisdom of Solomon, so long shall we, acting on the best opinion we can obtain, and which science shall give, commit errors which the science of the next day will say have been of the grossest description.'

(The Late Mr. A.J. Balfour in the House of Commons
May 11th, 1905)

'It is not reasonable to expect the higher forces to heal the infirmities of the body. Disease is brought about by the violation of nature's laws; hence the law demands obedience, and only through obedience unto the law will nature permit mankind to make good the wrongs imposed upon her.' — *(Dr. O. Ha'nish).*

(We would add that when a soul has faith, 'with God ALL things are possible', while remembering that 'faith without works is dead.')

'Wisdom resteth in the heart of him that hath under-standing.'

(Solomon)

ANCIENT AND MODERN RECIPES
FOR HEALTH AND HAPPINESS

Everybody should read the foreword before looking up the various subjects.

Those intersted in homoeopathy are strong advised to obtain a homoeopathic materia medica and repertory to learn more about this method of treatment. Such a work of reference should be in every home.

IMPORTANT NOTE

Since the publication of the first edition of this book Acts have been passed which restrict the sale of several remedies but this will not affect the usefulness of this work.

When a reader has no stock, or finds it impossible to obtain a remedy that is recommended, it will be found that the medicines suggested as alternatives will have a similar action and they can be employed with confidence.

It is suggested that the reader should consult a Homoeopathic materia medica and repertory when in doubt about the suitability of any remedy but we hope that the following list of prohibited remedies together with their suggested alternatives will be helpful.

Aconite to be replaced by Eupatorium Per., Ferr Phos or Absinthium.

Antimonium Tart by Allium Cepa, Eupatorium Per or Euphrasia.

Arsenicum Alb by China or Xanthoxylum.

Baryta Carb by Kali Mur.

Belladonna by Ferr Phos., Absinthium or China.

Cantharis by Xanthoxylum, Origanum or Berberis Vulg.

China Arsen by China.

Cocculus by Absinthium.

Colchicum by Iris Versicolor, Arctium Lappa or Sarsaparilla.

Conium Mac by Phytolacca or Kali Mur.

Crotalus Hor by Cinnamon, Ferr Phos or Nat Sulph.

Fluoric Acid by Calc Fluor.

Glonoine by Ferr Phos., Viscum Alb or Sambul.

Granatum by Cinnamon, Baptisia or Echinacea.

Helleboris Nig by Ceanothus or Lycopodium.
Hyoscyamus by Echinacea or Scutellaria.
Ignatia by Chamomilla or Scutellaria.
Mercurius by Kali Mur or Sarsaparilla.
Nux Vomica by Calc Phos., China or Chamomilla.
Psorinum by Iris Versicolor or Sarsaparilla.
Sabadilla by Allium Cepa, Euphrasia or Natrum Sulph.
Staphisagria by Cina or Absinthium.
Strophanthus by Cactus, Convallaria or Spartium.
Tabacum by Lobelia Inf.
Tantalum by Sarsaparilla.
Veratrum Alb by Viscum Alb.

Where several homoeopathic remedies are advised try one
at a time for a short period and make a change if necessary. If
a combination is considered beneficial this is clearly stated.

In a few instances a small difference will be noticed in the
doses advocated for some remedies given under different
headings. This is quite in order. Occasionally the dose advised
under a heading is the quantity that should be taken in the
circumstances mentioned; but no harm will result if the doses
of the same remedy are taken as advised elsewhere. For
example: In mental conditions calling for high potencies the
dose may be taken twice or three times — three times if you
feel sure that it is the remedy you require. Also, herbal
remedies and the quantities advised for these may vary, and
as they are harmless considerable latitude is permissible.

ABSCESS

An abscess is a localised accumulation of pus. It is a collection of morbid matter which the system seeks to throw off. There is always an impure state of the blood when an abscess forms, so the remedy lies in purifying the blood and helping the system to eliminate the local accumulation of poisonous matter.

Poultices have been used for clearing up abscesses for generations; also local fomentations. The old-fashioned bread poultice did some good work and is still as effective as some of the more modern treatments. Simply break up some bread and mix it with a little hot milk or water, and apply to the abscess as hot as can be comfortably borne. Renew, if necessary every few hours.

More effective poultices, especially in stubborn cases, and where there is much pain and inflammation, are those made with herbs such as Slippery Elm bark, Comfrey leaves or roots, or Marshmallow leaves or roots. Crush freshly-gathered Comfrey or Marshmallow roots and add a little powdered Slippery Elm bark. If the Elm is not obtainable use Comfrey or Marshmallow alone; or, use Elm only. Mix whatever is used with either very hot water or milk and apply to the affected area, using sufficient to well cover the part. Fresh Comfrey or Marshmallow leaves may also be cut up and applied as a cold poultice. Once the poison has been drawn off stop the hot poulticing, and apply fresh cold Comfrey or Marshmallow leaves, or simply dry covering.

Another very effective treatment is to apply mashed up raw Potato. This is also very suitable for wounds that will not heal. Always apply the Potato poultice cold and renew every few hours.

Full information respecting various poultices is given under that heading. On the whole hot poultices are better for abscesses, and cold Potato for healing infected wounds; but one may always employ Potato after a short course of hot poulticing to promote rapid healing. Potato has the virtue of attracting morbid matter and promoting the healing of bone and tissue.

A modern aid to speedy results is the employment of the Schuessler biochemic cell salts known as Silica and Calc. Sulph. Obtain these in tablet form from a reliable homoeo-pathic chemist. Use Silica 6x. The sufferer to take two tablets, dissolved slowly on the tongue, before meals three times daily. This form of Silica is absolutely harmless, and its action is to enable the system to throw off pus. It 'ripens' an abscess, so hastening the effect of any poulticing. After the pus has been well drained away Calc. Sulph. 6x may be used to promote healing. Dissolve two tablets on the tongue before meals after finishing with the Silica. Biochemic remedies are natural and harmless to the body.

If desired a herbal medicine may be taken instead of cell salts. For this purpose use either the fluid extract of Blue Flag or Yellow Dock (obtain from a herbalist). Dose: half a teaspoonful of either remedy in a little warm water before meals three times daily. Or, make a tea of the herbs. (See under the various headings). These herbs are harmless cleansers of the blood and can only do good.

ACACIA

Away back in history the gum of the Acacia tree was used medicinally for both internal and external use. It is nutritious and healing, and is often employed as an ingredient in medicines for coughs, fevers, diarrhoea and catarrh. This gum is also known as Gum Arabic. Dissolved in water it makes an excellent adhesive.

Acacia is an old remedy for applying to the sore nipples of nursing mothers, for which purpose it is most effective, and quite harmless to the baby. Apply a pinch to the nipples when necessary.

When the stomach is very weak, sore or inflamed Acacia makes an excellent healing food, which can be tolerated when other foods cannot be taken, when it not only provides nourishment but heals the inflamed membranes. It may be mixed with Slippery Elm or taken alone. A most satisfactory healing food may be made as follows: well mix a teaspoonful of powdered Acacia with one of powdered Slippery Elm and one of barley flour. Then blend this with either a teaspoonful of common brown sugar or pure honey. Then add slowly a cup of hot milk, water, or part milk and water, mixing thoroughly all the time. This forms a complete meal of itself. It is of great importance in all gastric troubles, indigestion, inflamed bowels, diarrhoea, fevers and general debility. A cup may be taken once to three times daily as required. Promotes sleep when digestive upsets cause insomnia, and is soothing to the nervous system. This food has cured advanced stomach and bowel disorders when other means have failed, and duodenal ulcers have cleared under its action when the food has been taken on its own three or four times daily for two weeks. The addition of Slippery Elm makes mixing rather difficult, and if there is much trouble over this, powdered Arrowroot may be substituted in the same proportion; or use one teaspoonful of Acacia, two of Arrowroot and one of Honey; such a combination being much easier to mix and practically as effective. Indeed, a teaspoonful of Acacia in hot water will of itself form a healing food. Those who like a little more taste to any of these suggested foods may add a pinch of best powdered Cinnamon to each cup. The Cinnamon adds to the value.

ACIDITY

It may seem strange that an acid such as Lemon juice is one of the best remedies for acid indigestion; yet it is so. Two teaspoonsful of fresh Lemon juice (not the bottled variety) in a small glass of hot water taken in sips two hours after a meal has 'worked wonders' in such cases. Or, put a teaspoonful of white Vinegar, or, better still, Apple Cider Vinegar, in a wineglass of hot water. Take a tablespoonful of this half an hour before meals, again fifteen minutes before meals and finally immediately before feeding — three doses in all. If the acid taste is much disliked add a little pure Honey.

Another remedy for acid dyspepsia is a saltspoonful of glauber's salts in a large tumbler of hot water sipped slowly half an hour before breakfast daily for a week or so. If acid

16 THE NATURAL HOME PHYSICIAN

remedies fail, try the biochemic salts. Rheumatic sufferers may
say that acid remedies will increase their rheumatism, but
stomach acidity is something different. In fact many rheumatic
sufferers have been cured by taking Lemon before or after
meals, or Apple Cider Vinegar with Honey (See the
headings).

It may surprise some to learn that nothing more than the
thorough mastication of ALL food will cure acid indigestion,
but it has happened over and over again. The Saliva secreted in
the mouth deals with the very first and essential process of
digestion, and when the food is well masticated the natural
chemicals in the saliva prepare the food for the next stage of
digestion in the stomach. If the food is not masticated there
is not sufficient saliva mixed with it, and further processes of
digestion in the stomach are held up, causing indigestion,
acidity and malnutrition. Most thin people would put on
weight if they did nothing more than feed slowly; likewise
the fat would tend to lose some. Of course, what one eats is
very important (See *Diet*). Swallowing one's own saliva after
meals is also helpful. An old cure for acid indigestion was to
chew a small piece of Liquorice root before a meal. Liquorice
is an ant-acid. One or two Liquorice sweets, known as
Pontefract Cakes, will have a similar effect; but Liquorice
does not act with all people. Try out the various suggestions
and employ the one that suits the individual case.

Yet another remedy is raw Potato juice. Mash up a raw
Potato, place in a handkerchief and squeeze out a teaspoonful of the juice. Take this in a little cold or warm water a few
minutes before feeding. Potato juice is also a good remedy
for rheumatism and gout.

Food made with Acacia Gum, Slippery Elm, Marshmallow,
Arrowroot or Comfrey root is also excellent for many
sufferers from acidity (See **Acacia**).

Here is an old herbal remedy for acid indigestion: Take
one ounce each of dried Meadowsweet herb and crushed
Dandelion roots, half an ounce of Peppermint herb and a
small piece of stick Liquorice. Simmer the whole gently for
fifteen minutes in three pints of water. Do not use an
aluminium pot; use enamel, iron, stainless steel or tin, and
keep the lid on to prevent the steam from escaping. Dose: a
wineglassful taken warm for preference (although cold will do)

a few minutes before meals, three times daily. After simmering strain off the liquid and bottle. Keep in a cool place. The quantity of Liquorice used may be varied to taste.

ACNE

This skin condition is very distressing to young people for it usually manifests just at the age when both boys and girls like to be attractive. It is mainly due to the chemical and glandular changes taking place in the system; yet, if the blood and constitution were truly healthy there would not be any acne.

The diet should consist of plenty of fresh fruits and salads. Rich and fried foods should be avoided, and pure Honey should replace sugar for sweetening beverages. Rubbing a slice of Lemon or cucumber over the face at night is often helpful.

Keep the bowels regular by taking the breakfast recommended for Constipation.

An excellent medicine consists of —

Red Clover flowers	½ ounce
Peruvian bark	½ ounce
Stinging Nettles	½ ounce
Boneset herb	½ ounce

Place in two pints of cold water (not in an aluminium pot) and bring slowly to the boil. As soon as boiling point is reached remove from the fire. Keep covered and allow to stand for half an hour. Strain. Dose: A wineglassful before meals three times daily. May be sweetened with plenty of Honey, or flavoured with Liquorice. This is an excellent formula for all blood and skin disorders.

ADENOIDS

From a homoeopathic chemist obtain little sugar pills of Agraphis Nutans 3x. This is potentised bluebell. The strong tincture is poisonous but in the homoeopathic 3x potency it is harmless. So ask for Agraphis Nutans 3x. This remedy has been successful in helping to clear many bad cases of adenoids. The dose is three or four of the little pills (which taste like sugar) taken as sweets three times daily before or after meals. If there are signs of improvement after two weeks carry on with the remedy; if no improvement, then bluebell will not cure.

Another proven remedy which may be tried is calcium iodine 6x. Give two tablets before or after any two meals of the day and continue for two or three weeks. This may be repeated later if necessary.

The child should be put on a cleansing diet, with sweet fruits and honey replacing sugar and the usual confectionery. Teach the child to perform this exercise for two or three minutes several times daily: Close one nostril by pressure with a finger and breathe in and out a few times through the other. Then do the same in reverse. Of course, in bad cases this is very difficult, and in such circumstances the services of a qualified practitioner should be obtained. If possible endeavour to find a cure without operation, as it sometimes happens that operative measures result in nasal troubles later on in life, although this is not necessarily so. (See also **Catarrh**).

AGAR-AGAR

This is a form of Japanese seaweed. It is soothing and nourishing, and makes a suitable jelly for invalids and those with weak stomachs. Agar-Agar aids bowel movement, but is very gentle in action and would appear to owe its action more to its 'lubricating' effect on the walls of the intestines than to any stimulating quality. A jelly is made by dissolving one ounce in about a pint of boiling water. May be flavoured with Lemon or prune juice. A teaspoonful of powdered Agar-Agar may be taken with soaked prunes for breakfast as an aid to the bowels in costive people.

AGE (Old) — (See under Rejuvenation)

AGRIMONY

This common plant is one of the best tonics growing on British soil. It belongs to the Rose order of plants and at one time held a great reputation as a remedy for indigestion, general debility and a sluggish liver. The old authority on herbs, Gerard, says: 'A decoction of the leaves is good for them that have naughty livers'. Agrimony is still very popular in France as a tonic beverage with meals; and it is also used as an application for sores, sprains and bruises, the bruised leaves being bound over the affected area. Pliny called it a herb 'of princely authoritie'. Agrimony promotes the appetite, tones the stomach and bowels, aids the function of the kidneys and is a mild but effective remedy for simple diarrhoea. In the old days it had a reputation for the treatment of constitutional weakness, probably because it aids assimilation.

In some respects its tonic action is almost equal to that of Peruvian bark, and is more acceptable to some people than the latter. For any of the troubes mentioned it may be taken as a tea or in the fluid extract form. To make a tea simmer an ounce of the herb in one pint of water (aluminium pots should not be used for boiling herbs) for fifteen minutes. Strain. Dose: half a teacupful before every meal. The dose for the fluid extract is half a teaspoonful in half a teacupful of hot water.

AIR BATH

The human skin is an important organ of elimination, and over-clothing is not a good thing. Most civilised peoples wear far too much on their bodies. We breathe through our skins, and every one of the millions of tiny pores is a sort of waste pipe for eliminating toxic matter in the form of wet or dry perspiration. When these pores become clogged skin elimination is held up and the extra work is thrown on to the kidneys. Likewise, when the kidneys are weak the skin takes over some of the work normally performed by these organs. That is a reason why sufferers from kidney complaints often have wet, clammy hands. Oxygen is also drawn into the organism via the skin, so it is obvious that a healthy skin helps to maintain bodily vitality. A vigorous skin also aids the circulation.

Some years ago a young boy was covered in gold leaf to take part in a carnival. He died and the investigation revealed that he had actually died from suffocation. The gold leaf had effectively sealed all the pores in his skin, and lung respiration had not been sufficient to keep the blood oxygenated. The Indian Mohawk chief, Os-ke-non-ton, told the writer about a party of white men, which included a doctor, who visited his tribe in Canada in the middle of a severe winter. The white men were muffled up to their ears to keep out the cold. The doctor in the party noticed an Indian brave standing in the snow with nothing on but a loin cloth. Said the doctor to the brave, 'Aren't you cold?'. The Indian replied, 'Is doctor's face cold?' 'No' responded the doctor, to which the Indian replied, 'Indian, him all face!'. Now, the doctor's face was the only part of his anatomy not smothered with furs, and the skin of his face alone was truly healthy. The Indian, by exposing his body to the air, had a healthy skin through which his system breathed and eliminated; as a result he had a good circulation. You will find that deep breathing exercises will warm you when you are cold (See **Breathing**).

Here we must sound a note of warning: do not suddenly leave off clothing to which the body is accustomed; leave some of the outer garments off gradually, and in the warm weather. When winter comes do not over-clothe again. Arctic explorers have discovered that wide mesh undergarments keep them far warmer than thick wool, and the reason is that the netting-like garments permit the air to circulate close to the skin. Do not be afraid of catching cold by wearing less — you won't. Rather, you are less likely to get chilled.

Daily air baths are a healthy habit. A good time to expose the body to air is during the morning toilet operations. Exercise is also better taken in the nude, and far more good will result. Running about in the nude, or near-nude, will also be very beneficial. One of the benefits of sea-bathing is the exposure of the body to air, and not all the value comes from the dip in the water. Air baths invite vitality of mind and body. Make them a daily habit.

ALCOHOLISM

Psychological aid is usually necessary, but we might discuss some remdies which tend to reduce the craving.

Angelica herb, taken as a tea, or in tincture form (See **Angelica**), three times daily, is claimed to have a desirable effect. Also homoeopathic Quercus 3. Dissolve three or four of the little pills on the tongue a few minutes before meals. If Angelica is taken as well, have this after meals. It is better to take each remedy for a trial on its own.

For alcohol poisoning there is no better remedy than

homoeopathic Ledum 30. Take three or four pills of this remedy on rising and again on retiring for about three weeks. Ledum 30. is quite harmless; it eliminates the poisons and is a remedy for many complains due to alcohol poisons in the system. These good effects have been achieved in a great many cases.

Alcohol is often a barrier to the healing of chronic disease, and it should be taken in strict moderation. However, a little wine before meals suits some people and is a digestive tonic. St. Paul told Timothy to 'take a little wine for your stomach's sake'. Brandy and whisky are given as stimulants (medicinally), but they are not so good as a few drops of tincture of Capsicum in hot sweetened water.

ALUMINIUM

A great deal has been written about the danger of using aluminium cooking pots, pans and kettles. The most careful investigation shows that this criticism is justified. Under the action of moist heat aluminium oxide contaminates both food and drink. This upsets some people more than others. It can cause digestive upset, catarrh, nervous disorders, intestinal trouble, mental disturbance and many other troubles.

There are those who, on the other hand, blame cooking in aluminium for almost every disease under the sun, which is sheer rubbish. Readers are advised to discard their aluminium cooking utensils and use glass, iron, stainless steel, tin or enamel. Of course aluminium looks very nice; so does a gold coated poison pill. Weakly folk with feeble digestions are especially warned against using aluminium in the kitchen. For more information read *Aluminium, A Menace to Health* by Mark Clement (published by Health Science Press).

Certainly all herbal teas should be brewed in pots which will not contaminate the medicine. Aluminium is likely to interfere with the remedial virtues of any herbal preparation.

ANAEMIA

Anaemia simply means poor quality blood. The blood of an anaemic person is not rich red; it is pale and watery. The cause lies in faulty nutrition due to digestive and assimilative faults. It is useless pointing to any one organ and saying that the cause is poor functional activity of that particular bit of mechanism, for several can be involved. One may say that organs mainly at fault are the spleen and red bone marrow. The red blood cells are manufactured (for want of a better term) in the marrow of the long bones, and the spleen is a blood reservoir. The stomach, liver, pancreas and small intestine may also be causative factors. Anaemia may be local or general. Local anaemia can be due to mechanical interference with the circulation in a certain section of the anatomy. There are various forms of general anaemia, ranging from the simple to leukaemia, which is a serious disease, and has been termed cancer of the blood.

It is useless 'feeding up' for the cure of anaemia, for unless the food eaten is assimilated no good will result. Much the reverse: the weak organs will be taxed beyond their capacity and the system become toxic, which only adds to the trouble. But the nature of the food eaten is most important. Anaemia sufferers should perform gentle deep Breathing exercises to increase the oxygen supply (See **Breathing**). Air and morning Friction baths are also most helpful (See under **Air Bath** and **Bathing**).

Yeast foods such as 'Marmite' or 'Yeastrel' are good for this trouble. Stale wholemeal bread, or rye bread, should replace white bread. Sugar should be avoided, and plenty of pure Honey taken instead, even for sweetening beverages. Fresh fruits, sweet dried fruits and well-masticated salads are indicated; but above all the food eaten must be very thoroughly chewed. (See **Diet**).

For a very long time orthodox medicine has prescribed iron tonics for the cure of anaemia, but the human body was not designed to feed on crude minerals. There is evidence to show that the excessive employment of iron as a medicine has actually brought about anaemia. Moreover, it ruins the membranes of the stomach and causes digestive troubles. It is now realized that iron is only one of the minerals required by the body in anaemia, and that it may take second place to calcium and sodium. Other minerals, known as trace elements, are also frequently indicated. If mineral remedies are given they should be in biochemic form (See **Biochemistry**). The sufferer may take two tablets of Calc. Phos. 3x before meals, and two of Ferr. Phos. 6x after meals. Also two of Nat. Mur. 6x on rising and again on retiring. A few weeks on this form of treatment may do a great deal of good. These biochemic minerals are harmless and are in the fine form in which they are found in the plant kingdom. They do not accumulate in the system and cause harm, but aid the body to assimilate their like from the food eaten, thus correcting assimilative faults.

Or, a herbal tea may be employed. Here is a tried and tested formula:—

Great Periwinkle herb	½ ounce
Wild Marjoram herb	½ ounce
Agrimony herb	½ ounce
Chamomile herb	½ ounce
Gentian root (in powder)	1 teaspoonful

Simmer the herbs in three pints of water in an iron or enamel pot for fifteen minutes. Keep the lid on and simmer very gently, as boiling takes away much of the virtue. Allow to cool before taking the lid off the pot. Strain. Then add one ounce of the fluid extract of Oats (Avena Sativa). If the sufferer has very poor circulation, add twenty drops of tincture of Cayenne (Capsicum) as well. Bottle, cork tightly and keep in a cool, dry place. Dose: a wineglassful before meals three times daily. Children less according to age. Remember that a bright and hopeful disposition is one of the best tonics possible.

ANEURISM

This condition calls for expert attention. Simple, effective remedies which give help and are not in any manner dangerous, are the fresh plant tinctures (obtainable from homoeopathic chemists) of Cactus Grandiflorus and Millifolium. Mix in equal parts. The dose is five drops in a little cold water before meals, three times daily. Also of value are the Schuessler cell salts Nat. Mur. 6x and Calc. Fluor. 6x. Take two tablets of Nat. Mur. 6x before meals, and two of Calc. Fluor. 6x after meals. Another good remedy is homoeopathic Baryta Carb. 12x. Dose: three or four of the little pills night and morning. Do not take all of these remedies together, but try the tinctures, the biochemics or the Baryta Carb. If one fails give the others a trial. The best plan is to get advice from a reliable homoeopath or experienced herbalist.

ANGELICA

This garden plant has considerable value as a medicine. It has been employed by British and Continental herbalists for generations as a remedy for indigestion, flatulence, kidney weakness, colds and as a tonic. Icelanders eat both the stems and the raw roots with butter. It is claimed to have some value in the treatment of rheumatism and gout. An ancient superstition was that Angelica was revealed in a dream by an archangel to cure the plague: hence its full name, Angelica Archangelica.

An infusion of the plant may be made by pouring a pint of boiling water on an ounce of the bruised root, or on the entire herb; the dose being two tablespoonsful before meals three times daily. It is certainly an excellent remedy for indigestion, especially when flatulence is present. Chewing the leaves, or a piece of the root, may have similar effects. The dose for the fluid extract is a small teaspoonful in warm water, but in the preparation of such extracts much of the value is lost. This is true of all aromatic herbs.

Homoeopaths claim that five drops of the strong (mother) tincture, three times daily, will produce a disgust for alcohol. Also, that it is good for giving tone to the organs in general and helps to cure indigestion, nervous headaches and bronchitis.

ANGER

In anger the face of one person will become red, and in another white. In the first instance the heart is forcing the blood to the surface, and drawing it inwards in the second. This shows how easily the emotions affect the circulation. But emotions do far more than that: they upset the nerves, interfere with digestion and poison the brain. Anger, for example, creats a deadly poison which plays havoc with mind and body. Most people 'work it off' by physical movement, yet some damage always results. Anger uses up a great deal of energy, and in this hectic life we need all our energies of mind and body to keep fit. To indulge in an evil emotion can so deplete the energy required for digestion that one may suffer stomach distress for hours or even days afterwards.

Anger is a form of fear, and fear is man's worst enemy. It is when we fear people that we get angry with them, although, of course, there can be other causes, even as there are different forms of anger, such as a righteous anger at evil-doing.

Those who indulge in evil emotions often do far more harm to themselves than to those to whom the emotions are directed. All the negative emotions of fear, hate, anger, jealousy and selfishness damage the system far more than wrong feeding. Regrets for the past, peevishness, envy, morbidness and 'nasty-mindedness' of all kinds are destructive in nature.

To overcome negative emotional states see the paragraphs under **Psychology** and **Spiritual Aid**. As a rule anything which helps the body aids the mind. One man, prone to anger, used to run to the bathroom and plunge his head into cold water when he had feelings of being overcome by his emotion. Others just take a walk. Certainly we may say that engaging in something physical will take the mind off incidents that tend to provoke anger. Of course it takes some will power to do these things, but that is what the will is for. All effort at self-mastery pays in the end by bringing a measure of peace, not only to oneself but to others. Frequently treatment by a skilled homoeopath will remove those subtle causes which produce temper and bouts of anger. The cause may lie in the gandular system, and there is nothing like homoeopathy to correct glandular disorders. For instance: an over-active thyroid gland will cause excitability and emotionalism. By normalizing the faulty gland the sufferer becomes more placid. One can do a great deal for oneself by mental control, but it is not easy when the glandular system is deranged. So, if one is conscious of his or her mental and emotional defects, a visit to a good psychologist or a homoeopath may produce a great deal of good. A sick liver will make one 'livery', morbid and disagreeable. Likewise a morbid mind can cause liver and stomach upset. Some writers stress the effects of mind over body rather much, forgetting the effect of physical disorders on the mind. The truth is that mind and body are of the one person, and it is the entire individual that needs attention.

ANGINA PECTORIS
This is a condition which calls for professional attention.

However, the sufferer can do much for himself, and cures have been accomplished in quite severe cases by the intelligent employment of harmless herbal or homoeopathic remedies. Angina is a very painful heart condition. It may be termed neuralgia of the heart, and can cause great fear and anguish.

By improving the circulation to the nerves from the spinal cord to chest and heart much relief can be obtained. To do this get a bowl of really hot water, and one of cold; also two towels folded so that they can be placed lengthwise along the spine. The patient lies face downwards as comfortably as possible in a warm room. Wring out a towel in the hot water and apply over the spine. This towel should be as hot as the patient can stand without undue discomfort. Cover with a blanket. After two or three minutes take off the hot towel and apply (gently) a towel wrung out in cold water. This towel should remain on for a minute or so. Take off the cold towel and apply a hot one for two or three minutes. Repeat this operation six to twelve times, finishing off with a cold application. This treatment may help a total cure if persisted with daily for some time.

Another method is to apply hot towels only to the spine (five or six of them, each remaining on for two or three minutes), and then giving some deep massage to the upper part of the back. Work the muscles away from the spine. That is, pull the tissues from the spine by using a sort of kneading movement. Skin polishing is next to useless; deep massage is necessary. Special treatment such as Chinese Acupunture sometimes produces totally satisfactory results in these cases.

Natural medicines have also cured Angina, even when orthodox methods have failed. One of the best remedies is the fresh plant tincture of Cactus Grandiflorus. Get this from a homoeopathic chemist, as the dried plant tincture is of little value, and few herbal stores stock the fresh plant preparation. As the dose is small it is necessary to purchase only a small quantity; say, one to two ounces. Dose: five drops in about a teaspoonful of cold water before meals three times daily. The treatment will be speeded up if the sufferer also takes two tablets of Mag. Phos. 6x after meals, three times daily. Severe cases may get better results by taking these remedies in homoeopathic potency. So, if the above fails get the same remedies in this form: Cactus Grandiflorus 30. and Mag. Phos. 30. The remedies will be in the form of tiny pills. Dose: three or four pills of Cactus Grandiflorus 30. dissolved on the tongue on rising, and three or four of Mag. Phos. 30. on retiring, i.e., one dose of each daily. Try either system of treatment for three or four weeks. However, it is wise not to let this treatment go on for long, and if there should not be any response to home treatment call in a reliable homoeopath. Dangerous drugs are quite unnecessary.

APPENDICITIS

We do not think it wise to advise home treatment for this trouble, as delay could be dangerous. On the other hand, the appendix is an organ performing a work for which it was designed by nature. Cutting it out does not remove the reason why it became inflamed, and the loss of the organ could result in toxic bowels later on. A skilled healer will give the best advice.

A pain in the region of the right groin which may or may not extend to the umbilicus (navel), associated with nausea, could be appendix trouble. Or it may be nothing more than old-fashioned tummy-ache. Hundreds of people have lost a healthy appendix through faulty diagnosis. It became the fashion in the reign of King Edward VII to cut out the appendix whenever there was a pain in this region. Doctors know differently these days.

If one gets pain and discomfort (without great distress) in this part of the abdomen the following medicine could be tried:-

Homoeopathic Dioscorea 30 and Baptisia 30. Take four or five pills of Dioscorea 30 before meals, and four or five of Baptisia 30 after meals, three times daily. If discomfort persists after two or three days have the condition diagnosed. Properly selected homoeopathic remedies have cured some of the worst cases of acute and chronic appendicitis, but treatment should be in the hands of an experienced practitioner.

Incidentally, do not take purgatives if you get severe pain over the appendix. Have no food, and take only weak Lemon or orange drinks. Wait for professional advice.

APPETITE

Over-eating of wrong, highly-seasoned foods will create a false appetite. The system calls out for certain nutrients, and when these elements are not present in the unnatural food eaten the body continues to call out for more and more food. This over-eating causes toxaemia (system poisoning) and leads to all manner of disease. Wholemeal bread is a real food which satisfies, while white bread is sheer rubbish. Natural food and sensible living will cure gluttony.

Sometimes an excessive appetite points to constitutional trouble which calls for investigation. Pancreatic weakness being an example.

In some cases homoeopathic Iodine 3 will regulate an excessive appetite. Take three or four pills before meals. But it all depends on the cause.

When the appetite is poor there is the same call for attention to diet and the habits of life in general. One may be sure of this: when the body does not want food it is utterly wrong to force food upon it. Only *wanted* food can be properly digested, and it often happens in cases of poor appetite that a short fast will prove to be a cure. Make no mistake, one will not die from lack of food. The remedies suggested for Anaemia are likely to improve the appetite. Whether appetite is poor or excessive the thorough mastication of all food is essential. (See **Diet**).

APPLE CIDER VINEGAR

This deservedly popular preparation is not a new discovery. Exponents of natural therapy have been advocating it for many years. Unfortunately it is regarded in some quarters as being a 'cure-all', and there is no such thing. Human beings differ so very much, and consequently their requirements with regard to food and medicine differ also.

Experience, which is the best teacher, shows that Apple Cider Vinegar does not suit everybody. It can upset some types, and accomplish no good whatsoever. Those who wish to try this remedy should take only very small quantities at first, and note the effect. It is often recommended with pure Honey. Here again, the addition of Honey agrees with most people, but not with all. The writer holds Honey in high esteem as a tonic-food; yet there are some people with whom it does not agree, although they are few.

Those who cannot take Apple Cider Vinegar may bring about a state of digestive trouble and anaemia if they persist in taking it because some authority has made great claims for its curative value. The rule is, if it does not seem to agree, cease taking it.

One or two teaspoonsful of Apple Cider Vinegar once or twice daily will do much to cure indigestion in many cases, especially if there is a sluggish liver. It is helpful for weak kidneys and cleanses the blood. Some rheumatic cases have been helped by this remedy, and a few have been made worse. On the whole it is suitable for those who wish to reduce weight. When there is nervous exhaustion add extra Honey to each dose. It should always be taken in water: one or two teaspoonsful of the Vinegar to half or three-parts of a tumbler of water. There are instances where this remedy will perform much good in the system for a time; then the good effects cease and there is some upset. When such a stage is reached do not take any more. This is true with every remedy under the sun. One can take too much, and for too long a period.

Try it for indigestion, sluggish liver, general debility, nervous exhaustion, bowel disorders, rheumatism, high blood pressure and obesity. A dose once or twice daily (preferably morning and night) is suggested. People who cannot take fatty foods may receive much benefit from this natural beverage, and even the thin will improve, provided it agrees with them.

ARNICA

In homoeopathic doses this is a wonderful remedy for fatigue and exhaustion, especially when due to over-work or to muscular strain. It should never be taken in its material form. Homoeopathically prepared it is quite harmless.

Arnica will very often remove all, or almost all, the consequences of falls, blows and injuries. Many years ago the writer had a patient who had been a very sick man for some twenty years. He had received a blow playing football, and had been knocked out for a few moments. He had never been the same since that time, and suffered from headaches, depression, indigestion and marked debility; he could work only for short periods. He was given one dose of homoeopathic Arnica in the 200th potency. The very next day he was better, and within a matter of two or three weeks was as well as he had ever been. Of course such astonishing cures happen very rarely, but when the right remedy to remove the cause has been administered such cures can and do take place. In this instance the concussion was the original cause of all the man's symptoms, and Arnica was the remedy.

When there is muscle strain, or any organ of the body is suffering from the result of strain or injury, Arnica may be tried. The inexperienced should not experiment with high potencies, but use the 3rd or 30th potency. Give three or four little pills of this 3rd potency before meals, three times daily. When quite certain of the cause it may be better to give a dose of Arnica 30 on rising, and again on retiring for a week or so, and note the results. If there is no improvement after two weeks, then Arnica is not the right remedy. Arnica 30 is excellent for mental and physical exhaustion, and for all sore, lame, bruised feelings and conditions.

The strong tincture is often applied locally for sprains and bruises, but *never apply Arnica to any area when there are abrasions, cuts or when the skin is broken.*

ARROWROOT

There are few curative foods to equal Arrowroot gruel for weakness of the bowels and diarrhoea. It is a natural tonic to the organs, and has been highly praised for generations. Boil two teaspoonsful in a pint of milk or water, or half milk and water, for a few minuts. Add Honey, brown sugar, Cinnamon or fruit juice to taste. The addition of Slippery Elm adds to the value. (See **Slippery Elm**).

ARTHRITIS

This distressing disorder is one of those always difficult to cure. Medical science has discovered possible cures from time to time, but they have never proved wholly successful, and in some instances make the sufferer worse. It is true to say that herbal and homoeopathic remedies have produced the best results; also plain, straightforward nature cure has proved helpful.

Attention to diet is essential (See **Diet**). Once or twice weekly take an Epsom salts bath (See **Epsom Salts**). Rubbing the body all over daily with domestic Vinegar is also of some service. Painful joints should be thoroughly massaged with Castor oil.

One of the best homoeopathic remedies is Silica 6 or 30. Try the 6th potency, and if no benefit after three weeks give the 30th a trial. Take four pills of Silica 6 before meals three times daily. The dose for Silica 30 is four morning and night. If Silica fails try Urea 30. Four pills morning and night. Other valuable remedies which may be tried are Guaiacum 6, Rhus Tox. 6, Bryonia 6, Urtica 6, Colchicum 6, and Ledum 6. Unless all symptoms are taken into account it is difficult to select the best remedy out of these six, but as a guide it may be said that Bryonia suits dark, irritable people who are thirsty and much worse when moving about. Those requiring Rhus Tox. are usually better for warmth and movement. This latter remedy is probably used more than any other homoeopathic medicine for the treatment of rheumatic ailments, but it does not give relief or cure to everybody. Colchicum or Guaiacum may be tried when the above fail to give relief. Urtica has produced excellent results, especially when irritation of the skin is present. Ledum seems to be one of the best remedies when the joints are much affected.

In all cases try Silica and Urea first of all, and give them a fair chance to act.

Here is a very effective herbal formula:

Fluid extract of Guaiacum	1 ounce
Fluid extract of Blue Flag	1 ounce
Fluid extract of Nettles	1 ounce
Fluid extract of Dandelion	1 ounce
Tincture of Cayenne	1 teaspoonful

Add the above to four ounces of cold water. The dose is one teaspoonful of the mixture in half a cup of hot water before meals three times daily. Also note the advice given under **Acidity**.

Herbal remedies are rarely nice to take, and the flavour may be improved by adding fruit juice, Honey or Liquorice, the latter being an excellent cover for bitter medicine. Molasses may also be used. Stinging Nettle tea has been known to bring about a cure. It should be taken regularly for some time. Simmer an ounce of the herb in a pint of water for fifteen minutes, keeping the lid on the pot. Dose: a wineglassful before meals. (See also **Rheumatism** and **Rubbing Oils**).

Employ rubbing oils if necessary, but never use these over swollen or inflamed joints.

Emulsified cod-liver oil is highly recommended by many practitioners. Add one tablespoonful of best cod-liver oil to two tablespoonsful of strained fresh orange juice. Use an electric mixer or plunger type mixer to well emulsify the oil. The more mixing the better. Take on retiring at least three hours after the last meal of the day. The preparation MUST be taken on an empty stomach. If desired take on rising instead of nightly, at least one hour before breakfast.

Some may prefer to use new milk instead of orange juice, in which case use two to four tablespoonsful of milk to one of the oil. Be sure to mix thoroughly.

After two or three weeks (longer in stubborn cases) take every other day for a time, and later on just once or twice weekly until clear of arthritis. The preparation may be flavoured with a few drops of essence of spearmint or peppermint if desired. The oil also supplies the iodine needed and vitamins A and D.

If the suggested dose seems to cause upset smaller quantities of oil may be used.

ARTIFICIAL RESPIRATION

The Holger Nielson Method is as easy as any to perform, and very satisfactory. Have the casualty face downwards with his arms folded so that his forehead rests on his forearms. See that the neck is fully extended. If available place a pillow or any available object beneath the folded arms to help keep the head up somewhat and tilted back. Then kneel by his head, placing one knee near the head and one foot by an elbow. Place the hands over the casualty's shoulder blades, with the thumbs touching the spine and the fingers spread out. Keep your arms stiff. Then rock foward gently and apply light pressure by means of the weight of the upper part of the body. Count mentally two seconds. This two-second pressure causes the casualty to breathe out. Rock backwards, gradually removing the pressure, and slide your hands to the casualty's elbows. Take about one second to do this. Then raise up the casualty's arms by his elbows until slight tension is felt. This movement takes two seconds. Then allow the elbows to return to the first position and again place your hands on his back. This movement should take another second. Repeat this rocking, pressure and elbow raising operation at the rate of about ten times every minute. The degree of pressure used depends of course on the casualty's age and sex, and when his or her arms are injured raise from the shoulders instead of the elbows. Always obtain professional aid as soon as possible.

Fresh air is essential, and people should not crowd round. Always see that there is no tight clothing about the neck.

Mouth-to-mouth breathing, or 'the kiss of life' as it is termed, is popular to-day, although it was first used by Elisha to restore the son of the Shunammite woman. (2 Kings 4:34). Lay the casualty on his back with head extended. Place one hand on the forehead and the other under the chin to tilt the head backwards. Open your mouth as wide as possible, take a deep breath and place your lips around his mouth. Then exhale into his respiratory organs. The hand that is over the casualty's forehead should be so placed that the fingers can pinch his nose to close the nostrils while the operation is taking place. Then remove your mouth, take a deep breath and repeat. Endeavour to perform the act at the normal rate of breathing.

Breathe more gently into the mouths of young children. With the very young your mouth can cover both nose and mouth of the child.

A series of sharp slaps between the shoulders will revive in some cases. Deal more gently with the young.

Valuable literature on first aid is supplied by the St. John's Ambulance Association and the Red Cross.

ASAFOETIDA
The powdered gum of Ferula Foetida is a natural antispasmodic. It is also slightly stimulating and has expectorant properties. It is one of the best of the old remedies for flatulence, especially in nervous subjects. It is doubtful if there is anything better for the dyspepsia of nervous, highly-strung sufferers. Hysterical flatulence usually responds to Asafoetida. A good pinch in a little hot sweetened water

before meals is suitable in most cases, but slightly more may
be taken if deemed necessary. For nervy, excitable children
make the dose a small pinch. Sweeten with Honey or flavour
with Liquorice.

In some cases this remedy acts better in the third
homoeopathic potency (Asafoetida 3). Dose: three or four
pills dissolved on the tongue before or after meals. Take on
retiring if there is insomnia due to flatulence.

ASPARAGUS

A garden vegetable that is very good for strengthening the
heart and kidneys. A medicine for weak or enlarged hearts is
made by mixing the freshly expressed juice with Honey and
taking a dessertspoonful three times daily. Heart and kidney
sufferers who eat the cooked vegetable will also receive a
measure of benefit, provided the cooking is done conservatively.

In some country places the roots of Asparagus are boiled
in water and the water taken in wineglassful doses as a
treatment for rheumatism. This is not very pleasant to take,
but the taste may be improved by adding a few drops of the
extract of Liquorice; or use Honey or Molasses.

ASTHMA

Simple cases of asthma have been cured by a short fast of a
few days on water or fruit juices only, followed by a natural
diet with a low starch content, plenty of fresh salads and the
avoidance of sugar. Sufferers should eat fresh Comfrey leaves
when in season with their salads. Gentle breathing exercises
are also most helpful (See **Breathing**).

Here is a reliable herbal medicine.

Hyssop herb	1 ounce
Lobelia herb	½ ounce
Grindelia herb	½ ounce
Cut Liquorice root	½ ounce

Place in three pints of water and simmer gently for fifteen
minutes, keeping the lid on. Use an iron or enamel pot.
Remove from the fire and add immediately one medium-
sized onion, cut up finely. Let stand until cool. Strain. Dose:
one or two tablespoonsful before meals, and again on

retiring, if necessary. Children less according to age. This medicine is harmless, but if it should cause nausea reduce the size of the dose. In some cases the value is further improved by adding to the above mixture, when cold, two tablespoonsful of malt Vinegar, or Apple Cider Vinegar. Keep the mixture tightly corked in a cool place. Hot towels to the spine followed by spinal massage, as outlined for the treatment of Angina Pectoris, is always very helpful in asthmatic cases.

Sufferers should take a deep, hot foot-bath for ten minutes nightly, as this helps to relax the system and equalize circulation.

As a rule asthmatic people are rather tense and inclined to be sensitive, especially to people and circumstances. A quiet mind is a great aid to ultimate cure.

Probably the best remedies are homoeopathic. Oleander 30 heads the list. Take four pills of Oleander 30 on rising and on retiring for two or three weeks. If results are not entirely satisfactory Lobelia 30 or Grindelia 30 may be tried in the same manner. Other good and proven remedies are Sambucus 30 and Belladonna 30. Note that Belladonna in homoeopathic potency is no longer a poison and is completely harmless.

Herbal or homoeopathic medicines may be tried, and if one fails the other should prove successful. The writer has cured a great number of cases with both methods, but always attention has been paid to diet and the habits of healthy living. Cardiac asthma calls for heart remedies, such as Lily of the valley.

Emetics give instant relief in most asthma attacks. See under that heading. Discontinue inhalers as soon as possible. They have caused many deaths.

AUTO-TOXAEMIA (SELF-POISONING)

The chief area from which the system is poisoned is the colon (large bowel). When there is constipation, toxic substances are retained and absorbed into the blood. This self-poisoning gives rise to all manner of diseases, hence the vital importance of having regular bowel action. (See **Constipation**). One may say that it is useless trying to cure any disease when one is being constantly poisoned from a costive state of the bowels. Indeed, one may lose his ailments once the body is clear of waste matter. The mind, too, benefits for the brain is nourished by the blood like all other organs, and pure blood makes for clear thinking.

Fasting, which is the animals' way to health, improves skin activity; deep Breathing, sane Dieting and right thinking — all help to cleanse the system of accumulated poisons. There are also some very effective remedies. But it must be remembered that the effects of remedies cannot last unless the basic causes are removed and those causes usually lie in wrong living and negative thinking.

The late Dr. Guyon Richards discovered that homoeopathically potentised Granatum was a most effective remedy for bowel toxaemia. Another is Sulphur and a third Echinacea. Granatum seems to suit most cases; but, if the sufferer has certain Sulphur symptoms, such as sensations of heat, burning and itching of the skin, a sinking feeling about 11 a.m., a dirty appearance and foul discharges, Sulphur is more likely to be the remedy. Try Echinacea if the above fail.

The method of dosage suggested is four or five pills of Granatum, Sulphur or Echinacea 200 on rising, and again on retiring. On the day following the doses of the selected remedy in the 200th potency, take the same remedy in the 30th potency. Four or five pills on rising and five again on retiring. Keep up the treatment with the 30th potency for three or four weeks.

Echinacea is also a satisfactory remedy in the form of fluid extract. Here is a reliable medicine in herbal extract form:

Fluid extract Echinacea	1 ounce
Fluid extract Yellow Dock	1 ounce
Fluid extract Blue Flag	1 ounce
Water	1 ounce

Dose: half to one teaspoonful in a little hot water before meals, three times daily. If constipated add half an ounce of fluid extract of American Mandrake to the above mixture. As a rule a laxative breakfast and the advice given under **Constipation** will make this added purgative unnecessary. Do without it if possible.

BABY

When baby cries look at the way he hold his fists. If the thumbs are held inside the fist the cause is internal discomfort. If his tummy is upset give him the medicine advised under **Teething**. If the thumbs are held outside the closed fists, then the pain is due to external discomfort; so look at the nappy, safety pins, etc.

BALM

Sweet, or Lemon Balm is a fine old remedy for stomach upset and simple feverish conditions, especially of children. Adults may find it of benefit; although, as it is so pleasant to take, it is most suitable for the young.

Place an ounce of the herb (fresh or dry) in a jar and pour on one pint of water that has boiled and allowed to cool slightly. Cover, and allow to stand until cool. Dose for stomach upset is a tablespoonful for young children, and a wineglassful for adults. Repeat if necessary. A pinch of Cinammon adds to the value, and the tea may be sweetened with Honey if desired. For feverish conditions, colds, etc., give young children a tablespoonful every hour, and less frequently as the condition improves. Adults to take a wineglassful in the same manner.

BARBERRY

The bark of the Barberry (Berberis Vulgaris) is one of nature's best gifts to mankind for digestive, liver and kidney troubles. It is helpful in the form of a tea or fluid extract, but the homoeopathic mother tincture is strongly advocated, as the results obtained from this are quicker and far better. Also, the dose is small. Barberry may be employed for all stomach and liver troubles, biliousness, and indigestion; also for weakness of the kidneys, gravel and difficult urination. It is also a fine remedy for gall stones. Experience shows that it is helpful in rheumatic ailments, probably owing to its toning and cleansing action on the eliminative organs. Its antiseptic properties make it a valuable medicine when the bowels are toxic.

Take five drops of the homoeopathic mother tincture in an eggcupful of cold water before meals, three times daily. Continue the treatment for three or four weeks, when all-round improvement should be noticed in the digestive system, kidneys and the general health. In some instances the 3rd homoeopathic potency acts better. Try taking five pills on the tongue three times daily, before or after meals. One advantage of taking this remedy in potency is that it is tasteless, this making it very suitable for children. The five-drop dose of the mother tincture may be sweetened with a little Honey if desired.

BATHING

Water was probably the first curative agent ever used by human beings. It has been employed for physical purposes during the known history of mankind, and finds its place in much spiritual symbolism, representing cleanliness of mind and freedom from sin. Examples are Christian baptism and the crossing of the Jordan.

When a Roman army encamped the first consideration was given to the baths, for they were their field hospitals.

During the last century there were several noted health homes in Europe specializing in hydrotherapy, which is the term applied to healing with water in the form of baths, showers, packs, etc. People flocked to these places of healing from all parts of the world, for they undoubtedly 'delivered the goods' and produced cures which were beyond the capacity of orthodox medicine to perform. Today, nature cure homes still use water treatments, and with marked success. The famous medicinal spas are still visited by the health-hungry, seeking new life and vitality.

No doubt, by making bathing a religious act the priests of old managed to get people to keep themselves clean and healthy; people who otherwise would have developed diseases due to filth and inactivity of the skin.

Water properly used, stimulates the circulation, and anything which improves the flow of the blood through the organism is bound to do good. Furthermore, bathing activates the skin and improves the condition of the blood. Read what has already been said about **Air Baths** and the importance of skin activity.

Cold and hot water may be employed for treatment purposes, and while we favour, in most instances, the application of cold water it must be said that hot applications also have their uses. Cold water, when applied to the skin, first drives the blood inwards; but, to quote a known law: 'action and reaction are equal but opposite'. Hence, after the first flow of blood inwards there is an immediate reaction, and the life fluid comes to the surface taking with it the toxic causes of disease for elimination through the pores of the skin. This reaction is kept up for some time, relieving congested organs and stimulating the organism. Hot water first draws the blood to the surface, and any curative action is speedy, although it does not tend to last. That is why rest is advisable after hot applications, while either exercise or vigorous movement should follow a cold splash. With cold packs, however, rest is also necessary, as we shall demonstrate.

While being enthusiastic over cold bathing and packs we cannot ignore the great value of hot applications in certain conditions, and also as a means for relaxing and softening up the tissues prior to manipulation. (See also **Epsom Salts**.)

Here are some ways of employing water for health giving and curative purposes.

FOOT BATHS

A really hot foot-bath before retiring is one of the best methods of helping to promote restful sleep. It relaxes the system and brings repose to the mind. Congestion in the head (a cause of insomnia) is relieved; hence the hot-foot bath is good for headaches and in cases of high blood pressure. Such a bath is also helpful for colds and chills. The sufferer should retire to bed immediately afterwards. When the hearing is affected by catarrh a hot foot-bath will sometimes do much to remove the obstructive cause. The hot water should reach well up over the ankles, and the feet should be bathed for about ten minutes. When drying pull the toes and twist the feet to loosen them up, as this adds to the beneficial effects.

Rheumatic sufferers may add a dessertspoonful of Epsom salts to the water, while those who have very sore and tender feet will benefit by the addition of a heaped teaspoonful of common domestic borax.

When a cold is threatened have a hot foot-bath, and at the same time drink a cup of Yarrow or Herbal Composition tea. Then get to bed, and the chances are that the cold may be aborted, or its severity greatly lessened.

FRICTION BATHS

To improve the circulation, brace the system and dispel that morning gloom, rub yourself all over with the wet hands, or with a wet towel. Dry vigorously, or dress quickly without drying. No, you will not 'catch cold' by dressing on a wet body, which is a very different thing from getting wet when clothed. The writer himself ceased getting winter colds when he had a quick cold morning friction and dressed without drying. The effect is quite a tonic. Of course, one may dry before dressing if this is preferred.

The following letter appeared in the London *Daily Mirror*:

'I was born in a small village. My family was very poor and I, who was pale and thin, always seemed to have bronchitis.

When I was seven, a schoolgirl I knew had pneumonia and I saw that she was getting many visitors, lots of presents. I had nothing so I decided to get pneumonia at any cost. While my mother was away at the village shop, I put my chemise in a bucket of cold water, squeezed it out as best as I could and put it on again.

I was dressed again by the time my mother came back.

I sat all that day waiting for pneumonia and finally went to bed still in that wet chemise. Eventually it dried on me. But still no pneumonia.

When I look back, I think my mother, who was always most particular about drying and airing clothes, would have died of fright if she had known.

But the funny thing is that though I was such a weakly child, I have hardly had a day's illness since — and I'm nearly seventy!'

Sufferers from catarrh, neurasthenia, sluggishness and general debility will benefit greatly from a morning friction. Many a neurasthenic will leave his neurasthenia behind in the bathroom if this morning rub is kept up for a time; or, better still, made a daily habit. Life is made up of habits, good and bad. Cultivate the good ones and add years to a happy life. An excellent time to perform breathing and other exercises is after a morning friction.

HEAD BATHING

When you are fed up, angry or have a fit of the blues, hold your head under a cold tap and change morbidity into hopefulness. It's as simple as that. Just a few do this instinctively. One man, whose wife was a constant nagger, prevented himself getting into a temper and doing violence by using the cold water head treatment. Probably others do the same thing. Anyway, holding the head under the cold tap, or dipping the head and face into cold water for a minute or so daily, will do far more for health than seems possible. There is no doubt that making a habit of this dispels mental and physical fatigue, tones the nerves, aids the circulation and improves concentration. It also tends to produce a healthy scalp and promotes the growth of hair. Unlike the friction rub, it is wise to dry the head thoroughly after this treatment.

HOT AND COLD PACKS

Cold water packs to cover the entire trunk, or the abdomen only, will do much to relive feverish conditions and draw out causative morbid matter from the system. In some health homes it is regarded as the best of all cures for fevers and auto-toxaemia (self-poisoning).

Cold packs should always be administered in a warm but airy room. A small sheet is wrung out in cold water and folded double. The sufferer is wrapped carefully in this folded wet sheet, and then covered with one or more dry blankets. The weaker the sufferer the more dry covering should be used. Always have a waterproof sheet on the bed. Weakly people should have a hot water bottle to the feet, especially in the winter. In some cases additional hot bottles may be placed on either side of the sufferer. The pack may remain on from one to three hours, according to the symptoms and the patient's comfort. As a rule sweating soon takes place. Some even go to sleep in a cold pack, and in such circumstances let the patient sleep on and remove the pack when he awakes. If a patient does not sweat within half an hour remove the pack and rub him well with warm Olive oil. One to three packs may be administered every twenty-four hours, according to the symptoms and requirements. In most instances the pack becomes yellow with the morbid matter drawn out of the body. All packs should be boiled after use. In the case of very weakly persons apply the pack to the abdomen only.

The abdominal pack is excellent for bowel disorders kidney weakness and female troubles. It is almost as good as the larger pack for feverish conditions, influenza, toxic states, etc.

Except in the case of very weakly people who react poorly to packs, sufferers should be sponged all over with Vinegar after treatment, and dried thoroughly. As stated previously; those who do not react by sweating should be rubbed over with warm Olive oil, and no further packs applied.

Hot packs may be applied to the spine or abdomen to soften the tissues and induce relaxation before massage or manipulative treatment. The method is described under **Angina Pectoris**. Hot spinal packs are excellent for reducing nervous tension and inducing sleep.

HOT LOCAL APPLICATIONS

Everybody knows the value of hot fomentations for painful areas, nerve pains and for treating localised septic conditions of the skin; but few know of the great help obtained by applying hot towels to the anus. This method is of great value when one is tensed up, irritable, exhausted and feels like passing out. The action obtained is probably through the nervous system. Those who are interested in Zone Therapy will realise the value of treatment to the anus when it is known that all the body zones are in that part of the anatomy. This treatment will also produce results when there is abdominal pain, and it will sometimes promote a bowel action. Hot towels should not be applied in cases of piles.

The sufferer adopts a squatting position, and has a bowl of really hot water and a small folded towel. The towel is dipped in the hot water and held to the anus. It should be as hot as possible without causing great discomfort or scalding. The towel is held in position for a minute or so, and the application repeated several times. The sufferer will shortly feel much better, when the treatment can be discontinued.

THE SALT GLOW

This is a morning tonic to the system which is superior to the ordinary cold friction bath.

Place a few handsful of common salt in a bowl and add just sufficient water to moisten it. Take up the wet salt in the hands and rub it all over the body. Swill off the salt with a sponge. This tonic treatment should not be taken by those who have a very tender skin, or by those suffering from skin disorders. Otherwise, its tonic action is quite marked if kept up for some days or weeks.

SEA WATER BATHS

Natural salt water has a tonic action on the skin, and helps the circulation. Get sea salt, which is packed especially for the bath, from any chemist and add this to the usual bath of water (tepid or hot). Sea salt is not just sodium chloride; it has other vital minerals in it, and it has been proved beneficial in cases of weak veins, flabby muscles, disorders of the skeleton and some skin disorders. A strong sea salt foot-bath is most soothing and healing to sore, tired feet. All chemists stock sea salt.

SITZ BATHS

Sitz (sit) baths are ideal for treating congested conditions in the abdomen and pelvis, and have done excellent work for female generative troubles. They awaken the organs, enabling them to throw off morbid accumulations, tend to normalize monthly periods, remove the cause of pain and have a general tonic effect. The alternate hot and cold method is advocated.

Have two small portable baths, one with hot water and one with cold. Sit in the hot bath for three minutes, and then change over to the cold bath for one minute. Keep the feet over the side. Repeat the operation four to six times, finishing off with the cold. Rub dry. The water in the hot bath should be kept as hot as the patient can manage in comfort, and a little hot water from a kettle added two or three times to keep up the temperature.

A single hot sitz bath can be very helpful for female period pain. Hot towels to the anus may also be satisfactory.

VINEGAR RUBS

Equal parts of vinegar and cold or tepid water rubbed over the body with the hands, or applied on a sponge have an excellent tonic effect. (See **Friction Baths**). These rubs are not indicated when skin diseases exist.

A cup of Vinegar added to the normal bath is invigorating and has a toning effect on the skin. It is said to help make the system resistant to infection.

FOMENTATIONS

Hot fomentations are soothing and healing; they draw out the causes of inflammation and promote healing. While ordinary hot water may be used, far better results will be obtained if a Chamomile infusion is employed. Add a small handful of Chamomile flowers to a pint of boiling water; if more water is required add more flowers. The Chamomile fomentation is excellent for nerve pains, neuritis, etc.

BAYBERRY BARK

This is one of the chief ingredients of the famous herbal Composition Powder. It is a powerful but harmless stimulant and tonic, which removes morbid matter from the stomach and bowels and helps to equalize the circulation. Bayberry is a wonderful cleanser of the system. It also has some value as a corrector of the liver. Useful for colds, chills and conditions of coldness.

Here is a remedy for colds and chilliness:

Yarrow herb	1 ounce
Powdered Bayberry	1 teaspoonful
Powdered Cayenne	¼ teaspoonful

Simmer in a good pint of water for ten minutes. Strain. Take a small teacupful, hot. May be repeated two or three times daily if necessary. Do not take this remedy hot if you are going out, but it may be taken cold. Sweeten with Honey, or add a little Liquorice to improve the flavour. For removing morbid matter from the stomach and bowels, clearing away catarrh and adding tone to these organs, take a tablespoonful, warm — not hot, just before meals three times daily. This aids digestion and is a good general systemic tonic. Will cure diarrhoea.

BIOCHEMISTRY (SCHUESSLER SYSTEM)

The writer has probably typed more pages on this method of healing than has any other living author. Those who wish to go into the matter thoroughly should obtain one of his books on the subject.* Here all that needs to be said is that the Schüessler system of Biochemistry is a natural method of supplying to the system the vital mineral salts that are essential to well-being. The mineral salts do not replace those found in foods, but enable the system to assimilate and utilise those minerals. The theory is that all disease is due to a disturbance or lack of one or more of the various mineral molecules, and that by correcting the disorganization, or making good the deficiency, disease can be cured. The minerals are prepared according to the homoeopathic system, and are rendered as fine, or finer, than in plant life. Some astonishing cures have been obtained by this harmless system of medicine.

Twelve basic minerals are employed, although of recent years other minerals (the trace elements) have been added. It must be staed, however, that for many years the original twelve salts have produced most satisfying results.

BLACKBERRY

Both the root and the leaves are one of the best remedies for diarrhoea, especially when children are the sufferers. An infusion is made of either the fresh or dried leaves or roots — one ounce being simmered for a few minutes in a pint of water. Sweeten with Honey to taste. The dose varies according to age, one teaspoonful four or five times daily will often prove sufficient for very young children, while adults may require a wineglassful. Blackberry infusion is also a tonic to the mucous membranes and strengthens the intestinal muscle.

BLACK CURRANT

Black currant tea is a very old remedy for colds and sore throats. Indeed, we doubt if any modern medicine surpasses it for throat inflammation. One way of making the tea is to

* *BIOCHEMIC PRESCRIBER* or *BIOCHEMISTRY UP-TO-DATE* published by Health Science Press

pour a pint of hot water over a heaped tablespoonful of really good Black currant jam, and adding the juice of a Lemon with some Honey. May be taken in tablespoonful or larger doses several times daily. Very good for coughs when the throat is much affected with mucous. Fresh Black currants may be used instead of jam when they are available. An infusion of one ounce of the leaves to a pint of water serves a similar purpose, and has a wider field of action, as it aids the kidneys and has marked value in most inflammatory conditions and mild fevers.

Today it is widely known that the Black currant is very rich in vitamin C, which is the blood cleansing, anti-cold vitamin. Black currant juice, *free from artificial preservatives*, is an excellent beverage for promoting the body's resistance to colds.

BLADDER WEAKNESS

A tried and proved medicine for weakness of the bladder and kidneys, gravel, etc.

Buchu	½ ounce
Uva-Ursi	½ ounce
Juniper berries	½ ounce
Couchgrass	½ ounce
Broom	½ ounce

Place in three pints of water in an iron or enamel pot, and bring slowly to the boil. Then simmer gently for ten minutes, keeping the lid on the pot. Allow to cool and then strain. Keep tightly corked in a cool, dry place. The dose is a wineglassful before or after meals. Honey or black treacle may be added if desired. The dose for children should be less according to age. This medicine has cleared up kidney and bladder trouble when the best medical attention has failed. It is ideal for urinary disorders in general, incontinence of urine, dropsy, gravel and stone. It is very soothing and healing to the organs and urinary passages. (See also **Runner Beans**.)

BLADDERWRACK

This sea plant is known as Kelp, and is one of the popular 'cure-alls'. The writer has to confess that he is one of those who has been guilty of praising this remedy; but, it is not a cure for everything and does little or no good in some cases. In others it seems to correct all manner of physical ailments, possibly due to its natural iodine content. One point in favour of Kelp is that it is one of the few natural remedies not contaminated by chemical sprays and poisonous fertilisers; although there is now the danger of our sea food being spoilt and rendered dangerous by radiation.

Originally, Kelp was chiefly used as a remedy for obesity; and here again its value in this respect is probably due to the iodine content acting on the thyroid gland. Yet, Kelp will also help the thin to put on weight, for it is a system *normalizer*. It has a beneficial action on almost every organ of the body and is good for endocrine gland troubles, nervous disorders, indigestion, poor assimilation, female disorders, liver congestion and sexual disturbances. Usually it aids the action of other remedies, and may be taken by all at any time, the only exceptions being those who get a little digestive upset from taking the remedy, and such are few.

Kelp is very rich in many vital cell salts (minerals) in addition to iodine, and supplies those elements lacking in civilized diet. A good way to take it is in powder as a condiment, lightly sprinkled over any food. Or, eat one or two Kelp tablets before meals. Homoeopathically potentised Kelp (Fucus) will work wonders in the hands of the skilled practitioner.

Kelp is claimed by some to act as a guard against some forms of atomic radiation — just one dose daily. The claim is, however, not proven.

BLOOD DISORDERS
Treat as for **Auto-toxaemia**.

BLOOD PRESSURE (High)
High blood pressure and arterial degeneration are very common, and wrong feeding has much to do with this. Sufferers should avoid all cooked and processed animal fats. Nut butters and margarines as supplied by health food stores are reliable, and the best cooking oils for sufferers are those produced from sunflower seed and maize. Cooked and processed fats and oils upset the liver, interfere with the body

chemistry and play havoc with the arteries. Avoid sugar and use pure Honey instead. Avoid table salt.

A tea made by infusing an ounce of Stinging Nettles in a pint of boiling water, and allowing this to stand until cool, will be very helpful. It tones the walls of the arteries and capillaries, helps to prevent capillary rupture (which causes strokes), cleans the arteries and helps to reduce blood pressure. Take a cupful before or after meals, and keep up the treatment.

Sufferers should also take plenty of fresh Lemon and Orange juice to supply ample vitamin P, which is an arterial tonic.

A really hot foot-bath at night is always helpful in these cases.

That type of blood pressure due to mental and emotional causes is best treated with herbs which have a calming effect, such as **Valerian, Scullcap** or **Chamomile.** (See the headings.)

Probably the best general homoeopathic remedy is Glonoine 30. Take the five pills morning and night for a few weeks, then have the pressure taken. continue with the remedy if improvement has taken place, which is very likely. The writer cannot recall a single case of blood pressure (except the nervous variety) which has not responded to Glonoine 30. But, if this fails one may try Aurum Mur. 30 or Viscum Alb. 30. (The same system of doses as for Glonoine). For nervous (emotional) blood pressure take Sumbul 30 morning and night for a time; or keep to herbal teas.

Those taking homoeopathic remedies may have Nettle tea as well if they wish, but do not take the tea within half an hour either way of taking the homoeopathics.

Sufferers from low blood pressure should follow the hints given under various headings for building vitality. The remedies suggested for **Anaemia** will produce results in such cases.

Rutin, a substance found in buckwheat, is rich in vitamins. It is stocked by most herbalists and health food shops. It's value has been well proven.

BLOOD TRANSFUSIONS

The transfusion of human blood both before and after operations and in certain constitutional conditions is very popular and much publicity is given to this satisfactory(?) method of saving lives and blood donors are praised for their services. Yet the public know very little about blood as a remedial agent, and still less about the other side of the matter — the possible harm.

Blood transfusions are not a new idea, but a very old one which has become common practice in modern times.

Keith Wheeler says that the diseases that lie hidden in human blood are extremely dangerous: syphilis, malaria, hepatitis etc.

The fact is that blood transfusion is a two-edged sword and danger lurks in every blood bank.

Every blood and tissue cell has its own life and this is part of the life of the individual, and this individual life contains all the positive and negative forces that make up the entity. Hence, when blood is taken from one body to another it carries with it the mental as well as the physical characteristics of the donor, the disorders that have not materialised and any mental state of an undesirable character.

There are records showing that in certain cases the character of a person receiving another's blood has been greatly changed, and not for the better.

Dr John Wallace states that 'Blood should be regarded as a dangerous drug.' He also says that 'there are now more than twenty viruses known to be transmissible by transfusion'.

Dr J.C.J. Ives, bacteriologist in Glasgow Royal Infirmary, revealed contamination of stored blood by cold-growing organisms, which he regarded as being extremely serious. He says that as little as 20ml. of blood can prove fatal.

Dr Philip Thorek, addressing over 1,000 doctors, said: 'I'm scared to death of blood.' He went on to say that 12,000 deaths were attributable to conditions brought about by transfusions in a single year.

Dr Herbert Ratner is reported to have said that more patients died from adverse reactions to blood transfusions than were saved by them.

Normal saline solution used instead of blood is quite satisfactory in most cases of surgery, even heart operations. No doubt a natural solution free from all danger will eventually replace blood.

Those who oppose blood transfusions on scriptural

grounds are not being more religious than scientific.

BLUE FLAG

One of nature's best blood cleansers. A fine tonic to the thyroid gland, liver, spleen and pancreas. In large doses it is a purgative. By far the best results are obtained when it is employed homoeopathically. For cleansing the blood and treating skin disorders the fluid extract may be used: half a teaspoonful in a little water before meals. For better action obtain the homoeopathic mother tincture of Iris Versicolor and take five drops in a little water before meals. Those who favour homoeopathy may try the 3rd potency in pill form, taking four pills before meals for impure blood, sluggish liver, thyroid trouble, spleen or pancreatic weakness. One may try this remedy when there are spots and pimples on the skin and when there is constipation, lassitude and that 'weak, out of sorts' feeling.

BOILS

Take the medicine advised for *Auto-Toxaemia.* Locally apply hot fomentations. See also under *Earth, Blue Flag, Poultices* and *Ointments.* Also various herbs. An outstanding homoeopathic remedy is Tarentula Cubensis 30. Five pills morning and night for a few days will usually clear up boils and eliminate septic conditions.

BONE DISORDERS

Comfrey tea is excellent for bone fractures to promote speedy healing. It promotes healthy bone growth.

Clubmoss (Lycopodium) is also helpful. Take five pills of homoeopathic Lycopodium 12 morning and night. Also two tablets of Calc Phos. 6x after meals, three times daily.

Comfrey tea may be taken in addition to other remedies. For preparation and dosage see under **Comfrey.**

BONE MEAL

The pulverised selected bone of cattle is now very popular as an accessory food for diseases due to a deficiency of calcium and other minerals. Undoubtedly, calcium in this form is acceptable to the body and is easily assimilated. There is evidence to prove that bone meal as provided by health stores and chemists has done a great deal for children suffering from rickets, anaemia and deficiency diseases. When there are bone disorders give a little bone meal with other food two or three times daily. Use the powder or take it in tablet form. One tablet two or three times daily is ample. Housewives may add bone flour to ordinary flour for bread and cake making. The entire family will benefit.

BONESET

An ancient remedy for colds, catarrh, fevers and lung weakness. Excellent for coughs, taken on its own or with other remedies. Boneset has proved to be a valuable remedy in influenza, especially when there is much aching in the bones and back. In all feverish conditions make an infusion of one ounce of the herb to a pint of water. Simmer gently for ten to fifteen minutes in an enamel pot. Strain. Take a wineglassful, hot, four or five times daily. For pains in the bones, without fever, take the infusion cold three times daily. Both the material doses and the homoeopathic form of Boneset (named Symphytum) have done much to correct disease of the skeleton, and it should be taken for poor bone development, rickets, brittle bones and disorders affecting the bones generally.

BRAIN FAG

Indulge in Breathing exercises. These cases need more and more oxygen. Also take steps to build up the system gradually. A hot-foot bath, or hot towels to the anus, will usually be very helpful when feeling extremely fatigued. (See also **Bathing**, etc.)

One of the best medicines is homoeopathic Kali Phos. 30. Dissolve four or five pills on the tongue morning and night for a week or two. Or take a herbal tea of Scullcap, Valerian or Chamomile.

BRAN TEA

This is another fine remedy for deficiency diseases, not only when there is a lack of Calcium, but when the body is short of iron, potassium, sodium, silica and other minerals. Pour a pint of boiling water over two heaped tablespoonsful of clean wheat Bran. Simmer for fifteen minutes. Strain. The

flavour is improved and the virtues increased if a handful of
raisins is added before simmering. Strain. Take a large
wineglassful, warm for preference, before meals. May be
sweetened with Honey. Lemon may be added to taste.

Give this tea daily to all weakly children and adults. Good
for anaemia, rickets, continual colds, catarrh, weak digestion,
sluggish kidneys, bronchitis and general debility.

BREAD

Bread has been termed 'the staff of life'. White bread may
be called 'the shackle of death'. A family of rats were divided
into two sections. One section was fed on white bread and
water only, and the other section on genuine wholemeal
bread and water. No other food was given. After a few weeks
those fed on white bread became ill and died. Those fed on
wholemeal bread were well and vigorous. Surely this speaks
for itself: the rats fed on the white bread were partaking of a
food almost totally deficient in mineral salts; hence their
organism gradually ceased to function. The feeders on
wholemeal were taking a food which supplied all the minerals
necessary to maintain good health. It is as simple as that!

The grain of wheat is a wonderful food, containing in its
germ and outer covering those vital elements which keep the
organism healthy and without which the life processes cannot
go on. On the other hand, white bread is lacking in these
minerals and is little better than a concoction of starch which
clogs the system, causes catarrh and supplies scarcely any
nourishment. Into the bargain the modern loaf is bleached to
make it the 'whitest white', and quantities of crude calcium
are added to the flour, which becomes a cause of many
ailments. People say that they can eat several slices of white
bread, but that they 'feel full' after eating much less
wholemeal. So they argue that they should partake of that
which they can eat most of. The truth is that the white
bread, being an incomplete food, cannot satisfy the body,
hence the need for more and more; while the wholemeal,
being a complete food, soon satisfies.

Bread should be genuine 100 per cent wholemeal, preferably made from wheat grown on composted soil. Such bread
will do much to eliminate illness and physical debility. White
bread is a curse. All wholemeal breads are good. Rye suits

those who tend to put on weight, and such are advised to eat the natural Swedish rye bread in biscuit form. Many cases of deficiency diseases have cleared up on a diet of wholemeal bread and fruit juices. Such a simple cure, but well worth trying when modern science fails.

'Give us this day our daily bread'. The good Lord supplies the ingredients; and, be it noted, bread is a Scriptural symbol of life — 'The bread of life'. Let us have this daily bread, but not the chemicalised, substitute of the shops.

BREAST TROUBLE (See Female Troubles)

BREASTS (See Female Troubles)

BREATHING

'God breathed into his nostrils the breath of life; and man became a living soul'. Genesis 2: 7. 'His breath goeth forth, he returneth to the earth; in that very day his thoughts perish'. Psalm 146:4.

The function of breathing is the very first and the last act of living. Man-made engines function on gas, chemicals, steam and atomic energy; the human engine functions on air. Air is just as vital to the human engine as steam, gas, etc., is to engines of metal — they cannot function at all without fuel. It follows, therefore, that an ample supply of oxygen-rich air is necessary to maintain the proper active functioning of all bodily organs; and air is indeed 'the breath of life'.

It is one of the major faults of human beings, especially the more educated, that they do not breathe deeply enough. In tests carried out by the writer it was discovered that about eight out of every ten patients registered an oxygen deficiency! Without enough of the gas which drives our human machinery, how can we expect to feel well or be radiant with vitality? We have known scores of people, weakly at one time, become changed beings through the daily practice of deep breathing exercises. Children, doing poorly at school, have thrived, become more mentally alert and passed their examinations; for oxygen is the one true food for the brain and better than any tonic. *Deep breathing will restore vitality, clear the mind and cure a large variety of diseases.* This statement is true and based on scientific fact;

but it is so very simple and not sufficiently complicated to satisfy the intelligence(?) of the average person, who wants to swallow health from a bottle. Of course breathing exercises take up a little time and the exercise of a spot of will-power; but is not the mind intended to master the body? Those who want radiant health must at least be prepared to give a little time to its attainment, for health is the greatest of all treasures, and life is sweet when one is well. Before we go further read what has already been written on **Air Baths**.

Deep breathing not only exercises the lungs, draws in more life-giving oxygen and stimulates the mind. The function causes the diaphragm to move as nature intended; this in turn gives a sort of internal massage to the organs of digestion, thus improving the digestion of the food and promoting normal assimilation. That is why fat people lose unhealthy weight, and thin people put on flesh, when they make a few minutes daily breathing exercises a habit. The heart is also strengthened and circulation improved. Most white people use only a small part of their lung capacity in the act of breathing, and the lungs are not one bit too small for the body they occupy. So exercise the lungs, get more life and really LIVE!

There is no need to strain at any breathing exercise; the lung function should be improved gradually, which is nature's way. Certainly sufferers from heart trouble and high blood pressure should make their exercises gentle, when no harm and only good will result.

BREATHING EXERCISES

1. One of the best, easiest and most natural of breathing exercises is to breathe to the rhythm of one's steps when walking. The most helpful breathing is when it is performed rhythmically — jerky breathing does little or no good. Walking puts rhythm into breathing. First, empty the lungs fully, and then breathe in gently and slowly as you count your steps. Commence with, say, four normal steps for the intake, pause for one step, and then count four for the exhalation; pause for one step, and then inhale again. After a little practice increase the rhythm to five for the inhalation and five for the exhalation, with one step pauses between. Then go on to six and, finally, to seven, which is the ideal rhythm.

In other words, as the normal step takes a second you will be taking in a seven-second breath and breathing out for seven seconds. Seven is the rhythm of life.

One very important point for all breathing exercises is correct posture. Hold the high high, the chin in, the abdomen drawn gently in and the chest out. Shoulders back and down. Do not adopt a stiff, military posture. If you hold the crown of the head high, the chin in and push the shoulders back and then allow them to drop, you will be in the correct position. Endeavour to confine breathing movements to the abdomen, as this is the proper way; and it exercises the diaphragm.

2. Stand or sit outdoors, or by an open window, in the correct posture, and breathe in for four or five seconds, pause, and then out for four or five seconds. Gradually increase the rhythm to seven seconds in and out as the lung capacity improves. One way of helping to maintain the correct posture is to bring the elbows back and place a cane or walking stick between the bends of the elbows so that the stick is across the middle of the back. Do this exercise for five to fifteen minutes once or twice daily.

3. When a cold is threatened it is often possible to abort it by concentrating on deep and prolonged exhalations. Breathe in and out fairly rapidly for a few breaths, then breathe in deeply and out slowly but very fully to thoroughly empty the lungs. Breathe out, without strain, until you cannot breathe out any more. Pause for a few seconds and then fill the lungs again. Take a few more rapid in and out breaths, and then repeat the exercise several times. Several people known to the writer have aborted colds by doing this, and the writer himself eliminated an attack of influenza by doing this for almost two hours! That is a long time, but it worked! *Whenever distressed breathe out deeply.*

4. To stimulate the mind when fatigued reverse the process. Breathe in and out a few times; breathe out fully and then in slowly and deeply to thoroughly fill the lungs. Hold the indrawn breath for several seconds, and then exhale. Repeat the process several times.

As a rule the lungs fill themselves if they are emptied to the degree nature intended, the filling being automatic. It is like squeezing a rubber bulb: when the air is expelled the bulb fills because it must. The same with the lungs. That is why we rather stress the importance of exercise No. 3 if the lung function is very poor. But there is never any need to strain. In the ordinary way exercises 1 and 2 are all that are necessary to build better health.

5. Another good exercise is to walk up the stairs breathing out. Take a few deep breaths, then one deep exhalation, walking slowly up the stairs while exhaling. Pause when the lungs are empty. Take a deep breath, and continue with a prolonged exhalation while ascending. This exercise has been known to tone up weak hearts, although those with heart trouble must never over-do it. Performed gently and gradually it will tone the heart muscle.

BRONCHITIS

Stubborn cases of bronchitis are often associated with a tendency to asthma; so in chronic cases, the treatment advised for Asthma is recommended. For ordinary bronchitis this herbal medicine will be of service:

Hyssop herb	½ ounce
Elecampane root	½ ounce
Elder flowers	½ ounce
Horehound herb	½ ounce
Powdered Ginger	1 teaspoonful

Simmer gently in two pints of water for fifteen minutes, and keep the lid on the pot. Allow to cool. Strain. Dose: a tablespoonful to a small cupful three or four times daily. Give the size of dose according to age. The medicine may be flavoured with a little Liquorice, which also adds to the medicinal value.

Another excellent remedy is prepared by melting one ounce of medicinal stick Liquorice in a pint of hot water. Then add four ounces of best Honey and a medium size Onion, cut up finely. Stir well, and allow to stand for an hour. Strain, and add a tablespoonful of Cider Vinegar or good malt Vinegar. Stir again. The dose for very young children is one or two teaspoonsful every hour or two hours; give a tablespoonful to older children, and a little more to adults. This preparation is excellent for coughs of all types.

Attention should be paid to the back as well as the chest. Wear red flannel over the back from the upper part of the hips.

The patient should remain in bed in a well ventilated room. The back should be sponged with hot water, dried and then gently rubbed with hot vinegar. Dry the back again and rub in warm olive oil.

In severe cases apply a hot bran poultice to the whole of the upper back. The sufferer should lie on his back on the poultice for as long as convenient. Renew the poultice if necessary. More than one is rarely required.

At the same time as applying the poultice, or even if no poultice is used, cold cloths applied to the throat and chest and renewed when they get warm, will help and relive any tickling.

Also most helpful is the administration of about three tablespoonsful of hot water every ten minutes for four hours (Prof. Kirk). This is also good for coughs.

After attacks weakly subjects should resort to the back protection mentioned above until the system has built up.

Rubbing the chest and back gently with turpentine is helpful in many cases of respiratory trouble.

BROOM

One of the best old herbal remedies for dropsy and urinary troubles. Tones the organs, regulates the water in the system and strengthens the heart. This simple herb has succeeded in producing good results in cases when orthodox medicine has failed; and it is harmless.

An infusion of one ounce of Broom tops to a pint of boiling water, allowed to stand until cool, is given in small wineglassful doses three or four times daily. Sweeten with Honey if desired. One may use the fluid extract instead of the infusion — half a teaspoonful in a little hot water three or four times daily; we regard the infusion as being superior to the extract.

BRUISES

Distilled extract of Witch Hazel is a good application. Arnica is also a fine remedy (See under **Arnica**). For bruised bones round the eyes (black eye) homoeopathic Ledum 200 is said to have excellent effects. Two doses of four pills; one on rising and one on retiring.

BRYONIA

This is one of the best medicines for rheumatism in cases where the sufferer is much worse for moving about. It suits people with dry mucous membranes, parched mouth, dry, stuffy nose, etc. Try the 3rd homoeopathic potency: four pills before meals three times daily. Most cases respond better to the 30th potency: four or five pills morning and night.

Homoeopathic Bryonia is also excellent for dry coughs, and is one of the best known medicines for pneumonia. For the latter we suggest a dozen pills of the 30th potency dissolved in half a tumbler of cold water, and the patient given a teaspoonful in minute sips every two hours. However, in these cases expert professional aid is advised.

Bryonia is not advocated in any form other than the homoeopathic.

BUCHU

A tea made from the leaves is a reliable herbal remedy for all urinary troubles. Infuse an ounce of the leaves in a pint of boiling water. Allow to cool. Give a small wineglassful three or four times daily for kidney and bladder weakness, gravel, catarrh of the organs. Or employ the remedies suggested for Bladder troubles.

BUCKBEAN (OR BOGBEAN)

A very old cure for debility, rheumatism and skin diseases. Infuse an ounce of the herb in a pint of boiling water. Allow to stand until cool. Dose: two tablespoonsful before meals three times daily.

It will be noted that several of the herbs mentioned in this book are for similar ailments. This is an advantage, for when one is not available, another can be used with every confidence.

BURDOCK

This is a wonderful herb for disorganised blood and nervous irritability. We have known it clear up the most obstinate skin disorders. Also, it has been successful in calming distressing abdominal conditions – pain, tension, gas accumulation – when other remedies have failed. It also acts as a tonic to the kidneys. The root or herb may be used, or the seeds. We suggest an ounce of either the root or the herb simmered gently in a pint of water for ten minutes, and allowed to cool. Strain. Dose: a wineglassful before meals three times daily. Burdock is a most valuable herb to have in the home. The fluid extract may be used if desired — half teaspoonful doses in hot water; but the infusion is better.

BURNS

A mash of scraped Potato applied to burns is very effective. Another treatment is to stew Marigold petals in a little water until they form a soft pulp, and apply cold.

Spearmint is excellent. Obtain the essence of Spearmint (not the oil). If this is not obtainable use essence of Peppermint. Sprinkle the essence over the burn or scald and keep the part exposed to the air. There will be smarting, but this passes away rapidly. As the pain returns sprinkle with more essence. Repeat at intervals until all pain has gone. If you have no essence apply finely chopped Mint or Peppermint leaves as a dressing. When treating face burns with essence keep the eyes closed. Marigold ointment is also fine for burns. Moistened salt applied to burns will prevent blistering; but it has to be applied quickly.

Urtica Urens (A Nettle used by homoeopaths) is most helpful used as an ointment, and also internally. Apply the ointment as necessary, and to promote healing from within take five pills of Urtica Urens 3 every hour for four doses, and then before meals three times daily. Obtain the ointment and pills from a homoeopathic chemist.

A compress of distilled extract of Witch Hazel is excellent for first degree burns.

When possible the immersion of a burned member in *very cold* water immediately following a burn, for fifteen minutes or longer, is excellent and it is as old as the hills.

Applications of grated fresh onion with a little salt added prove to be both soothing and healing. But keep in mind that severe burning calls for speedy professional attention.

CAJUPUT

Cajuput oil may be employed on its own, or in lotions in combination with other oils, for rheumatic and nerve pains, toothache, sprains and bruises. It enjoys an excellent reputation as a liniment. It may also be taken internally, although it is a very strong remedy and the dose is one or two drops only, on sugar. Used internally for spasmodic pains, flatulence, colic and whooping cough.

CAMPHOR

Camphor has been praised by herbalists, homoeopaths and orthodox physicians. Nobody seems to know exactly how it acts in the system, and even the great founder of homoeopathy. Hahnemann who knew more about Camphor than anybody else, confessed that he was puzzled by this remedy. But it certainly has a profound action on the system. It is of great value in the treatment of colds, fevers, fainting spells and hysteria. It has probably saved many lives and given speedy relief to thousands of sufferers. The action is very quick, and it is not intended to be used as a constitutional medicine over long periods. It is an *emergency remedy*. It may also be used as a lotion for rheumatic pains, neuralgia, gout, etc., although it is unlikely to cure such conditions; it does, however, bring relief. Embrocations containing Camphor have been employed successfully for generations. Useful for inflamed tissues, muscular pains, bruises, etc.

For internal use obtain Spirit of Camphor. Any chemist can supply this, but the best is that sold by homoeopathic chemists. The dose is one or two drops on sugar, or in honey. For emergencies, in heart failure and cases of shock, give such a dose every five minutes until a reaction takes place. Then cease giving the remedy. When a chill is threatened and the temperature is sub-normal, give a dose every fifteen minutes — three to six doses. Camphor is wonderful for cholera. As soon as the patient has reacted and the circulation established, just give a dose three times daily until well; or put the sufferer on other indicated remedies. Camphor will usually abort a cold very quickly if given at the very first signs of trouble; but if not given promptly it is practically useless. In such cases rely on suitable herbal teas. Even to smell Camphor will revive many who feel faint and who are in danger of collapse.

A fine remedy for weak hearts and sluggish circulation can be prepared as follows:

Fluid extract of Hawthorn berries   2 ounces

Fluid extract of Cactus Grandiflorus   1 ounce
Fluid extract of Fennel Seed   1 ounce
Tincture of Camphor   10 to 15 drops

Dose: about ten drops in a little warm or cold water before or after meals three times daily. This strengthens the heart muscle and valves, and is most helpful when the heart is upset by flatulence.

CARAWAY SEED

The seeds have been used as a flavouring and medicinal agent for hundreds of years. They strengthen the organs of digestion and are very good for flatulence, heart-burn, colic, abdominal pains and heart distress. Infuse a teaspoonful of the seeds in a pint of hot water and take a wineglassful when required. Or, take five to ten drops of the fluid extract in hot water. Sweetened with Honey and taken in smaller doses it is excellent for infants and the stomach upset of older children.

CARDAMOMS

The medicinal value of these seeds is similar to that of Caraway, although more greatly favoured by the profession. Probably the best way to take this remedy is in the form of Compound Tincture of Cardamoms; obtainable from herbal stores and chemists. The preparation has been used for many years as a remedy for digestive upset, flatulence, heart upset due to stomach derangements and acidity. A very grateful, warming and comforting remedy, and so pleasant to take. The dose is a teaspoonful or more when required, in hot water.

CASCARA

Cascara in fluid extract or pill form has been used for constipation with much success. It is also helpful in rheumatic disorders. The trouble with all laxatives is that in time they weaken the intestines, and larger doses have to be taken to produce effects. It is quite possible to cure constipation by diet alone. When the bowels are very obstinate Cascara is a satisfactory remedy which is not too habit forming, to be taken until the bowels move normally. A good preparation is made by adding one ounce of the fluid extract of Cascara to two ounces of Compound Tincture of Cardamoms. Dose:

half to one teaspoonful taken on retiring. Use a little more if necessary.

For rheumatism, piles, indigestion, sluggish liver and sick headaches this is also a very reliable medicine, although for such disorders the dose should be either five drops of the fluid extract or half a small teaspoonful of the mixture with Cardamoms (as above) before meals. Pills may be taken instead of liquid, although they are rather hard on the stomach. The liquid is to be preferred.

CASTOR OIL

Castor oil is usually regarded as nothing more than a strong purgative, and it may be used in essential cases for this purpose — one to four teaspoonsful at night, followed by a drink of lemon. But the oil has other uses. Some ladies of fashion have discovered that it is one of the best applications for skin blemishes, wrinkles, etc. It is gently massaged into the face on retiring, and is probably much better than the high-priced fancy, skin-clogging creams. It is also good for ringworm and irritable patches on the skin. Used as a massage oil it is excellent for rheumatic joints, and the writer almost always recommends his arthritic patients to use it for this purpose. Massage the affected joints for a few minutes twice daily.

CATARRH

This troublesome complaint is due to wrong feeding, and especially to an excess of starch and sugar. Sufferers should have more fresh salads and fruits, and replace sugar with pure Honey.

Juniper berries	½ ounce
Angelica herb	½ ounce
Peppermint herb	½ ounce
Sundew herb	¼ ounce
Powdered Ginger	1 teaspoonful

Place the herbs in two pints of boiling water and allow to cool, keeping the lid on the pot or jar. The dose is a wineglassful three times daily. For children a dessertspoonful to a tablespoonful according to age. May be sweetened with Honey.

The herbal remedy for Bronchitis is also quite good; or, the Liquorice and Onion recipe under the same heading.

Breathing exercises and morning Friction Baths (See **Bathing**) will do much to eliminate catarrhal conditions. We have known homoeopathic Calc. Carb. 30 clear up some very bad cases. Take four pills morning and night for a week or two. For thick, stringy catarrh of the nose, throat and bronchial tubes try Kali Bich. 30 morning and night for a while.

A stuffy nose can be cleared by using powdered Bayberry bark. Obtain a length of cycle valve tubing. Dip one end in the powder and insert *that* end in the nostril, then blow through the other end of the tube. Repeat with other nostril. This is excellent for colds and even for adenoids and thickening of the nasal tissue. Children with stuffy noses will sleep much better if the nose is cleared in this manner at night.

Cinnamon will sometimes cure catarrh when other remedies fail.

CATNEP

Catnep, or Catmint, is used for colds and fevers, and is similar to other herbs recommended for such conditions. It produces free perspiration, and the sufferer should go to bed after taking a dose. Infuse one ounce in a pint of hot water and allow to stand. Keep it hot, but do not simmer. Keep the steam from escaping. The dose for adults is one to two tablespoonsful, taken warm. Repeat every three hours. Give children one or two teaspoonsful, sweetened.

Many herbal practitioners advise a bowel injection of this infusion. Administer at blood heat, and be certain it is not too hot. Retain for as long as possible (the entire pint or less) before evacuating. Experienced practitioners say that it acts better for colds and fevers taken in this form. Also, this Catnep injection is ideal for inflamed and toxic conditions of the intestines. Experience shows that a daily injection for three or four days will do much to rid the system of poisonous matter.

Catnep tea is also useful for flatulent dyspepsia, and has a mild tonic action.

CAYENNE

Cayenne pepper (Capsicum) is a pure, natural stimulant. It will often aid the action of herbal teas when a good pinch or more is added to each dose. Authorities claim that, as a stimulant, it is superior to brandy, and experience suggests that this is so. Taken in hot water it removes obstructions, increases bodily heat and equalises the circulation; hence, it is a good item to add to remedies for colds.

Some of the old herbalists used to administer teaspoonful doses, but we think this is too much and over-stimulating; although a strong dose may save life when a powerful stimulant is called for.

As a tonic for the heart and circulation, and when one feels faint or a cold is threatened, take a quarter of a teaspoonful, or a little more, in hot, well-sweetened water. It will replace brandy at any time, and will do more good. Cayenne is also better to use as a condiment than ordinary pepper. Never use white pepper; use Cayenne or genuine black pepper. Cayenne will often help in the treatment of indigestion, especially when the digestive trouble is due to feeble stomach action. It is an ingredient in Composition Powder.

CELANDINE (Greater)

We advise this homoeopathically for liver disorders when there is a pain under the right shoulder blade. (The homoeopathic term for this herb is Chelidonium Majus). In such cases it rarely fails. Take four pills of the 3rd potency after meals.

CELERY

A very good vegetable for the nerves, and for those who suffer from rheumatism and fibrositis. A fluid extract of the seeds is more powerful than the raw vegetable. This also has a tonic action on the stomach and kidneys. Dose: five to ten drops in hot water before meals. If desired, purchase the powdered seed from herbal or health food stores and use as a condiment. Very good results should be obtained.

CENTAURY

A herb for improving digestion and increasing the appetite.

Centaury has been used for generations as a stomach medicine. It also has some value as a strengthener of the heart. Infuse one ounce in a pint of boiling water. Allow to stand for half an hour. Dose: a dessertspoonful to a wineglassful, sweetened, before every meal. Harmless and good.

CHAMOMILE

One of the very oldest remedies for indigestion, nervous trouble of all kinds and neuralgic pains. It is ideal for hysteria, and is most valuable for the nervous affections and period troubles of females. Infuse one ounce of the flowers in one pint of boiling water. Cover, and allow to stand for half an hour. Dose: one to two tablespoonsful three or four times daily; or when necessary. A valuable remedy for nervous headaches. Chamomile Flowers make a fine poultice or hot fomentation for nerve pains.

The homoeopaths employ the German Chamomile. Four pills of Chamomilla 3 before meals will do much to cure neuralgia, nerve pains, hysteria, irritability, nervous heart trouble, indigestion and bowel disorders. Some cases do better by taking the 30th potency once or twice daily. Chamomilla 3 is excellent for the nervous and stomach upsets of infants and young children. A remedy par excellence for Teething troubles. The little pills may be dissolved in the feeding bottle and taken with the feeds.

CHAPS AND CHILBLAINS

There are many good remedies for internal and external use. As a rule the main cause is a deficiency of calcium in the system, and two tablets of biochemic Calc. Phos. 3x or 6x, three times daily, will prove helpful in all cases. Also, take two tablets of Silica 12x every night.

There are excellent homoeopathic remedies for taking internally: Agaricus 6, Tamus 3, Plantago 3 and Euphorbium 6. All sufferers are advised to take Calc. Phos. and Silica, but to hasten results one of the homoeopathic remedies should also be taken. The selection depends on the general symptoms, and for this information it is necessary to look at the details of the remedies in a homoeopathic repertory. But no harm will be done if one remedy is tried; and, if that fails, one of the others. We suggest Tamus or Euphorbium. Try each remedy for a week or two: four or five pills a few minutes before or after meals, three times daily.

For external treatment Tamus or Plantago ointments (from homoeopathic chemists) are good. Apply two or three times daily. Or, massage the area with Compound Tincture of Myrrh (from herbal stores). Another method is to paint unbroken chilblains with Friar's Balsam at bedtime. Sometimes two or three applications will effect a cure. Yet another treatment is to bathe the areas with hot water in which potato peelings have been boiled. Twice daily is enough; and it is claimed that results are obtained quickly.

CHESTNUT

The leaves of the Chestnut tree have long been regarded as one of the best medicines for spasmodic and whooping coughs. There is ample proof that scores of bad cases of whooping cough have cleared up more quickly under its influence than would otherwise have been possible.

One ounce of the leaves are infused in a pint of boiling water, and allowed to stand until cool. The dose varies from a teaspoonful for the very young to a small wineglassful for adults, taken three or four times daily. If possible give a dose after a fit of coughing or vomiting.

CHICKEN POX

Boneset	½ ounce
Scullcap	½ ounce
Pennyroyal	½ ounce
Powdered Rhubarb	1 teaspoonful

Place in two pints of cold water in an iron or enamel pot, bring slowly to the boil and allow to stand, without further boiling, for half an hour. A dessertspoonful to a tablespoonful every two hours, according to age. Sweeten with Honey or flavour with a little Liquorice. Better given warm.

Keep the sufferer warm in a well-ventilated room. The less food the better, but give plenty of hot Lemon and Honey. Dab any irritable skin patches with distilled extract of Witch Hazel, and cover any bad pustules with linen saturated with the extract. Renew fairly frequently.

CHICKWEED

The leaves of this common garden weed are nourishing and healing. They may be added to salads for general benefit to the health. Powdered dried Chickweed is almost as good as Slippery Elm as a food for weak stomach and debility. Very useful in fevers as it is nourishing and so easily digested. Or, blend with an equal part of Acacia or Slippery Elm. Mix with a little cold water or milk, and some pure Honey. Then add warm milk gradually, mixing thoroughly all the time.

Chickweed ointment (obtainable from herbal stores) is one of the best applications for many skin disorders, itching and for sores about the eye-lids. Chickweed as a medicinal infusion, or as a gruel, is recommended for chronic rheumatism, indigestion, sluggish liver and lassitude.

CHINESE HEALING

The Chinese system of diagnosis from the pulse must not be confused with the modern method of pulse taking — it is very different and complicated. By this method the skilled operator can discover which organs of the body are affected. There are few Western practitioners of any school of medicine competent to diagnose by this method, which goes back for four thousand years; some writers say for longer.

The Chinese method of treating disease by Acupuncture and Moxibustion is gaining ground in France and Germany, although only a very few British medical men are interested. By both methods certain points on the skin are treated by the insertion of gold, silver or steel needles, or by slight burning. The methods are not nearly as painful as one would imagine, and quite often the needle prick is scarcely felt. These focal points on the skin act on the internal organs by stimulating or reducing the activity of the vital force as the occasion demands, through a reflex action. There are various views as to how and why the action takes place; but it certainly does. Our modern Zone Therapy is an example of obtaining reactions through the treatment of certain zones in the anatomy.

The writer was initiated into Acupuncture some time ago, and has achieved results thought to be impossible in various deeply-seated disorders. However, it is hardly a subject for the layman; and having mentioned its potency, we shall not discuss the subject further.

CHOKING

If this takes place whilst eating, thrust the finger briskly to the back of the throat to cause vomiting. When a fishbone is lodged in the throat suck a lemon, the juice of which softens the bone and helps in its removal. When there is a fit of choking, loosen the clothing and raise the victim's left arm above the head.

CINNAMON

Used in the East as a medicine for hundreds of years. It is one of the biblical medicines. Research work in Radiesthesia suggests that it has no equal in the vegetable kingdom in the treatment of toxic fevers, especially influenza. It acts well in both material doses and in homoeopathic potency. For home use we suggest the rubbed-up bark, or the powder. Cinnamon kills the 'flu virus, cleanses the bowels, reduces the fever without suppression and gives strength to the organism. A quarter of a teaspoonful in a little hot, sweetened lemon, taken every hour, is ideal for influenza. See also the method advised under that heading. A pinch of Cinnamon to a quarter-teaspoonful in water, Lemon or milk before meals, will aid digestion, dispel gas, tone the stomach and purify the bowels. Quite nasty painful states of the intestines have cleared up under the action of this medicine. It is an ingredient in Compound Tincture of Cardamoms, and also in the famous Composition Powder. Sometimes, Cinnamon is all that is necessary to cure a cold.

CIRCULATION (Poor)

Build up the system with Friction baths, Breathing exercises and sensible dieting. If the heart is weak see under **Heart.** If the system is toxic see also **Auto-toxaemia.** Composition Powder is a good general remedy; also Cayenne and Cinnamon.

CLOVES

Powdered cloves also find a place in Composition Powder. Cloves are warming, stimulating, aromatic and antiseptic. They help to clear away the toxic ground which favours the presence of streptococcus and staphylococcus bacteria, and destroy the latter. A good pinch of powdered Cloves in hot, sweetened water will eliminate flatulence and aid digestion, especially after eating fatty foods. Cotton wool impregnated with oil of Cloves is still one of the best remedies for an aching tooth, when placed in the cavity. The oil may also be used instead of the powder for stomach upset and flatulence — one or two drops in brown sugar or Honey. We regard the powder as being better for this purpose.

CLUB MOSS

This is the Lycopodium of the homoeopaths, and it has little value until it has been triturated by the homoeopathic method, when it becomes one of the most powerful yet harmless medicines for many disorders. Astonishing cures have been achieved with Lycopodium. It is exceptionally good for a weak stomach with digestive disorders, sluggish liver, malnutrition, kidney troubles, intestinal weakness, sexual disorders, aneurism, heart and aortic weakness and melancholy. While it does not always follow, the patient most likely to respond to this medicine is thin and has a dried-up appearance. The 12th or 30th potencies may be tried. Four or five pills dissolved on the tongue morning and night for two or three weeks.

COFFEE

Coffee is a nerve and brain stimulant, and too much of it produces nervous tension, insomnia and indigestion. Weakly, nervous people should refrain from it. On the other hand a small cup of black Coffee just before a meal will stimulate digestion, and in some instances can be taken with advantage for short periods. As Coffee over-stimulates and causes insomnia, the same item in homoeopathic potency becomes one of our best remedies for this trouble. Try four pills of Coffea 3 before meals for a time. If not very effective try the 30th potency: five pills on retiring only. Should results not take place within two weeks abandon the remedy as it will not be the one to meet the individual requirements.

COHOSH (Black)

Five to twenty drops of the fluid extract in a little hot

water before meals is good for coughs, diarrhoea and
obstructed menses. It has much value in the treatment of
rheumatism. As it has a direct action on the adrenal
(energy-creating) glands, it is a fine remedy for exhaustion
and general debility. For the latter, however, it is best taken
in homoeopathic potency: four or five pills of the 30th
potency morning and night for two or three weeks. May be
repeated if necessary. An excellent medicine in either form to
help women during the change of life.

COHOSH (Blue)

Similar to the above, but more especially a female remedy.
Used by Indian women to aid child-birth. Like the black
variety it is excellent during the menopause. Doses as for
Black Cohosh.

COLCHICUM

This is the Meadow Saffron. We recommend it only in the
homoeopathic form, when it is one of the best remedies for
rheumatism. It also acts on the sensory nerves and helps in
painful conditions of the muscles. If the rheumatic sufferer is
greatly prostrated, cold and has a sensation of electric shocks
in the body, is worse at night and from moving about,
Colchicum may be tried for a while. Four or five pills of the
3rd potency before meals three times daily, or five of the
30th potency morning and night.

COLDS

A cold is an eliminative effort on he part of the body to
throw off accumulated waste products and toxins. We are
always elminating through the skin, and when the outer skin
is chilled, or function is poor due to imperfect circulation,
the inner skin (mucous membrane) takes on the task. If the
system did not eliminate toxins by means of catarrh, then
other processes would be employed, such as a fever (burning
up process). The point is that colds, unwelcome and
distressing as they are, are nature's way of spring cleaning a
toxic organism, and but for this cleansing effort deeply-
seated conditions and some form of chronic disease would
take place. A good circulation and a healthy skin usually
mean freedom from colds. Do not suppress the cold, but aid

nature in throwing off the cause. As one wit has put it: a cold is both positive and negative — sometimes the eyes have it and sometimes the nose! Continual eliminative colds are debilitating, and the cause must be removed.

In spite of all the discoveries of medical science, a certain cure for colds has not been discovered. Yet the old herbalists have managed to clear up such conditions in quick time by using simple herbs. The application of Wet Packs over the trunk or abdomen are also most helpful (See **Bathing**). Also Turkish or sweat baths, provided one does not take a chill afterwards.

Here is a remedy that will take care of any cold — there is nothing superior:

Yarrow herb	½ ounce
Elder blossom	½ ounce
Peppermint herb	½ ounce
Cayenne pepper	1 teaspoonful

Simmer gently in an iron or enamel pot in two pints of water for twenty minutes, keeping the lid on the pot. A teaspoonful or more of Composition Powder may be used instead of the Cayenne, and if the cold is accompanied by fever use Cinnamon for preference. For children it is advisable to add a little Liquorice to disguise the flavour.

Take a large cupful and go to bed, with a hot bottle to the feet. Repeat in two hours if necessary, and again the next day. Always take it hot. Children less, according to age. Do not take this medicine hot if going out, as it causes sweating and another chill may result. But for a very mild cold a small cupful may be taken cold if the sufferer *has* to venture outdoors. Whether out or in bed, do some deep breathing. (See **Breathing**). It is wise to fast during a cold, taking hot Lemon and Honey only. If food is taken it should be very light and easily digested; such, for example, as Slippery Elm gruel. Man is the only animal who eats when he has a bad cold. (See also **Onion**).

Cinnamon, the great influenza remedy, will also prove most effective in clearing up colds and nasal catarrh. We have known it succeed in the most stubborn cases of continual colds which would not yield to other remedies.

In 'The Journal of the American Medical Association' it is

stated that those who are sensitive to cold can cultivate immunity by immersing a hand in *very* cold water for one to two minutes for three to four weeks. This gives systemic or general desensitization. The immersions should take place once daily, preferably in the morning.

COLIC

Outstanding remedies for colic are homoeopathic Colocynth and Dioscorea.

Five pills or five drops of Colocynth 6 administered every fifteen minutes will usually prove effective after three or four doses. If this fails try Dioscorea 3 in the same manner.

Those subject to colic should take Dioscorea 3 before meals three times daily for two or three weeks.

Dioscorea is usually known as Wild Yam by herbalists and those preferring herbal preparations should take half a teaspoonful of the fluid extract in a cup of hot water, this taken in sips, will usually give almost instant relief. It may be repeated in two hours time, if necessary. Honey or brown sugar may be used for sweetening.

Another good medicine is Herbal Antispasmodic drops which can be obtained from herbal vendors. The dosage is given on the label.

Those who favour the Schuessler cell salts should dissolve about ten tablets of Magnesium Phos. 3x or 6x in half a tumbler of hot water, and take a dessertspoonful in sips every fifteen minutes.

COLLAPSE

Hot Towels to the anus; Camphor or Cayenne as medicine. (See **Bathing, Camphor, Cayenne**). Get the sufferer to bed; and, if in doubt, seek professional aid. Composition Powder taken in hot, sweetened water is also a great restorative. See also homoeopathic **Arnica**.

COLOUR AND HEALTH

Colour plays a greater part in promoting health and happiness, or depression and misery, than is realized. It has even been recorded that certain debilitated and unhappy people have become more vital and radiant by changing the colour schemes in their homes.

Colour has been used therapeutically for a very long time, and it has been proved that by exposing sufferers from certain disorders to selected colours marked curative effects have been obtained. Some institutions employ colour rays by means of slides for this purpose.

Attention is drawn to the remarks given under **Gems (Curative)** and **Laws of Correspondence.**

One can have too much of any colour. It has been noticed that people living in homes where the decoration scheme has been predominantly red tend to become over-stimulated, excitable and prone to fits of anger. In a home where blue is over-emphasized one may find depression and morbidness.

The writer had one experience of a very debilitated and morbid-minded lady living in a home where the wall paper and even the drawing room furnishings were deep blue. She loved the colour; but after a time she was wise enough to change her colour scheme and became a different person without any medicinal aid.

COLTSFOOT

An old country remedy for coughs of all kinds, and very reliable. Simmer an ounce of the leaves in one-and-a-half pints of water for half an hour. Add a piece of medicinal stick Liquorice and dissolve. Dose: a large wineglassful three or four times daily. A little Cinnamon or Ginger may be added with advantage.

COMFREY

Comfrey leaves have general medicinal value cooked, or added to salads. They are nourishing and healing to the lungs and bodily organs generally. The roots have a much stronger action. Comfrey root infusion is a remedy of excellence for congestion of the lungs and coughs of all kinds. It is also a fine remedy to promote the healing of fractures; hence the old country name of 'Knitbone' for this plant. Comfrey heals and tones the mucous membranes of all organs; aids greatly in healing internal ulcers and tissue damage. If Comfrey is boiled with pieces of meat, you will see that the meat joins together, which is visual evidence of what it does to lacerated bone and tissue. This plant is receiving much attention from orthodox medical scientists, who have the most pleasing things to say about it. We anticipate that the main healing ingredient, which is already known, will be isolated, given a fancy name and sold at a high price. But the isolated element can never be the same as it is in its natural association within the plant as provided by nature.

Comfrey should be grown in every garden. Recently a skilled herbalist recalls that he was visiting friends in the middle of a severe winter. Snow was on the ground, and it was bitterly cold. The child of his friends was suffering from a severe, obstinate cough, which no remedy had touched, although several had been tried. On being told that Comfrey was in the garden, he took the necessary tools, broke up the frozen earth and managed to get a piece of Comfrey root. He washed it, shredded it, added hot milk and the child was given a desertspoonful or so of the Comfrey-impregnated milk every two hours. The cough had gone within twenty-four hours!

Freshly gathered Comfrey leaves are very effective for relieving and curing bronchial asthma. When in season they should be added to salads; and asthma sufferers should chew the leaves four or five times daily. In this respect the virtue of fresh Comfrey has been rediscovered, for it was held in high esteem as an asthma remedy generations ago.

Comfrey is highly recommended for disorders of the skeleton, defective and crumbly bones, bone decay, etc. It seems to be equally valuable in material or homoeopathic form. To make an infusion place half to one ounce of the fresh or dried cut up root (fresh for preference) in one quart of water or milk. Boil gently for about fifteen minutes. Strain. Give a desertspoonful to a wineglassful, warm, every two hours for coughs and acute lung troubles. The size of dose varies with the age of the sufferer. To promote the healing of wounds, ulcers and fractures give three times daily before meals; also for building the constitution.

Bruised Comfrey leaves applied to the affected parts are of great value in local wounds, swellings and inflammations. May be added to any poultice to improve the healing virtues. Additionally, Comfrey is one of the finest garden fertilisers.

COMPLEXION
True beauty comes from within; it can never be plastered

on. The rosy face and clear skin of a healthy girl puts any artificial complexion to shame. Beauty is also a state of mind. There are cases on record of women with pasty complexions and faces lined with worry who, by changing their thinking and cultivating happiness, have become radiant in face and personality.

From the physical standpoint, the first step to beauty is to get the blood healthy. This means Breathing exercises, Friction baths and a good bowel action daily. It means sensible feeding and living. Creams and powders, no matter how expensive or attractively packed, usually tend to ruin a complexion rather than improve it. These chemical applications clog the pores, interfere with the circulation and tend to deaden the skin. Frankly, women are fools to spend so much money on worthless concoctions, although we admit that there are a few creams that are free from bad effects and do what they are supposed to do — at least in a measure. Actually, oils are better than creams, but the oil should be thin for preference. Sweet almond oil is very good massaged into the face at night, but pure Almond oil is expensive and the substitute will not do. However, it costs less than many of the advertised creams. New milk is also excellent for the face. As a rule creams containing Witch Hazel have some virtue.

The way to obtain a natural complexion and rosy cheeks is to wash the face with warm water, and then finish off with cold. Dry thoroughly, and massage in some new milk or sweet Almond oil. If the face is dry, flabby or wrinkled use a slice of cucumber or Lemon instead of oil or milk. Keep up the treatment. Some ladies have obtained good results with Castor oil, and this is certainly effective in some cases. Another good application is the inner skin of peaches or apricots. We often hear the expression, 'A complexion like peaches'. Why not use peach peel and obtain such a complexion? Just rub the inner side of the skin over the face a few times, and don't wash afterwards.

Some authorities say that soap spoils the complexion, and the soda in most soaps is certainly not helpful. In this connection it seems necessary to advise a soap made in Ireland. We refer to M'Clinton's. Use the plain or the perfumed. This soap is free from soda and is of itself a complexion treatment. Unfortunately, it is difficult to obtain in some districts. Professor Kirk of Edinburgh has high praise for M'Clinton's soap, and advocated its use for general massage purposes, packs, etc. Failing M'Clinton's use Slippery Elm soap from health stores or herbal vendors.

Internally, a tea made from freshly gathered green Violet leaves and rose petals is unquestionably good for the blood and skin. Simply place a handful of either, or a mixture of both in a jug. Pour on a pint of warm (not hot) water. Allow to stand for an hour. Take a wineglassful before meals. Make freshly daily.

COMPOSITION POWDER

If the herbal profession had done nothing more than provide this powder for treatment purposes, it would have accomplished something worthy of the highest praise. The formulae vary somewhat, but the main ingredients usually consist of Bayberry, Prickly Ash, Cinnamon, Cayenne, Ginger and Cloves in suitable proportions.

The powder is supplied by all herbal stores and some chemists and it is not expensive. It may be taken alone, or added to herbal teas for the treatment of chills, colds and fevers. Also of value in cases of indigestion and general debility, toxaemia, etc.

The dose is from a quarter to half a teaspoonful in hot milk or water, sweetened with Honey or black treacle to taste. For colds and fevers take before going to bed. Taken strong it will help the system to sweat out the cause of the cold or fever. Continue to take a dose three or four times daily until well. Do not take it hot if going out, but a small dose in cold or tepid milk or water may be taken in such circumstances. For general constitutional weakness, indigestion, etc., take a small or moderate dose before meals, warm. Children, of course, require smaller doses than adults. See also Anti-spasmodic Drops under **Spasmodic Troubles.**

CONSTIPATION

This is the underlying cause of so many ailments ranging from self-poisoning in the intestines to rheumatism and general debility. Many sufferers cannot expect to get truly fit under any form of treatment until the bowels work normally.

Chronic constipation of years standing has been cured by diet alone, and mainly by partaking of a laxative breakfast. For example: have a plate of soaked prunes with some cereal, such as 'All-Bran'. The prunes should not be boiled, but soaked overnight in a teacup of hot water, or milk and water, in which half a teaspoonful of genuine Molasses has been dissolved. Molasses activates the bowels, tones the system, gives help generally to the constitution and aids in the elimination of rheumatic disorders. Agar-Agar, raisins, dates, etc., may be taken as well if desired. No bread with this meal. The beverage should be Dandelion Coffee (from health food stores) or a glass of hot water.

In obstinate cases Hot Towels to the anus may promote an evacuation. It is most important to adopt the Native Squat (see **Native Posture**), as this greatly aids the bowel activity, pressing on the abdomen and distending the anus. Several cases of severe constipation are known to have been cured by adopting this posture for evacuation. Of course it does not help right away, but will gradually achieve its purpose after being habitually practised for some time.

A short, sharp walk before breakfast encourages bowel movement. All body bending and twisting exercises are helpful.

Very bad cases may call for the use of an enema for a time. It is even necessary in an emergency to give a dose of Castor Oil. The use of purgatives should be gradually discontinued, as they only weaken the already debilitated bowels. Countless thousands suffer from chronic constipation as a result of taking purgatives instead of living sensibly. However, advice should be given to the unwise as well as to the wise, and the former, if they must take laxatives, are advised to employ herbal teas or vegetable pills.

Avoid mineral laxatives and medicinal paraffin. The latter, although not absorbed into the blood, coats the lining of the intestine and interferes with the absorption of nourishment from the food eaten, thus producing deficiency diseases and weakness.

Here is a harmless non-poisonous remedy that is not habit forming: Pour a good pint of boiling water over an ounce of Agar-Agar and a teaspoonful of Linseed. Simmer for five minutes. Take one to two tablespoonsful of the jelly formed before meals. This preparation may be flavoured with Lemon juice before it cools. A teaspoonful of powdered Agar-Agar may also be added to the laxative breakfast described above. Just sprinkle it over the food. Psyllium is a harmless laxative (See **Psyllium**).

Here is a laxative medicine that is effective; but, as with all purging medicines, it is advised for short periods only.

Fluid extract of Barberry	1 ounce
Fluid extract of Dandelion	1 ounce
Fluid extract of Cascara	1 ounce
Fluid extract of Liquorice	½ ounce
Tincture of Ginger	½ ounce

The medicine may be made more pleasant if two ounces of Compound Tincture of Cardamoms is added instead of the Ginger, although it will be somewhat weaker in action. Dose for the mixture: half to one teaspoonful in hot water at night. If Tincture of Cardamoms is used take somewhat larger doses.

A tea made from Senna Pods is also effective, and not unpleasant to take. Those who feel they must rely on pills can take 'Bile Beans'. These pills are about as good as any laxative of this nature can be. Other harmless remedies which act without purging are biochemic Nat. Mur. 6x before meals, and Nat. Sulph. 6x after meals. Or, homoeopathic Hydrastis 1x before meals. Get the latter in liquid form and take four or five drops in a little water. Other good homoeopathic remedies are: Opium 6. or Podophyllum 3x. Obtain these in pill form and take four of either before meals. These remedies cannot harm, and in order to select the best it is wise to consult a homoeopathic repertory. However, when one fails, the other can be tried. We favour biochemic and homoeopathic remedies, and diet with exercise, etc. In the name of sanity do not resort to the habitual use of purgatives as they lead to weakness, disease and constipated minds.

CORNS AND BUNIONS

Tie a fresh slice of Lemon over a corn, allow to remain on all night and repeat nightly. This will usually remove even bad corns. Another method is to paint the corn with homoepathic Thuja ∅ night and morning. Lemon is also helpful bound round bunions. The chief cause for both corns and bunions is tight shoes. Women suffer far more than men from these troublesome and painful offenders, and the reason is obvious — pride! Shoes of sufficient width and with reasonably low heels will ensure strong feet and good posture (See **Posture**).

To lightly dab corns with peroxide of hydrogen three or four times daily will often cause the corn to dry up. Another method is to apply a small pad of Castor Oil over the corn and keep it on all night, renew nightly until the corn comes away.

A little animal wool placed between the toes will be of much comfort when soft corns are present. A wad of animal wool placed between the great toe and the one next to it will also relieve bunions and help to straighten the toe. Do not use cotton wool as it becomes hard; animal wool retains its elasticity. Animal wool is often better than special rubber toe-separators.

For soft corns wrap a piece of soft linen soaked in turpentine round the toe. Keep on all night. Relief is speedy, and the corn will clear after several treatments.

COUGHS

Read the information given under **Asthma**.

Hyssop herb	½ ounce
Linseed	½ ounce
Boneset	½ ounce
Horehound	½ ounce
Elder blossom	½ ounce
Stick Liquorice	½ ounce

Place in two-and-a-half pints of cold water in an iron or enamel pot, and slowly bring to the boil. Simmer gently for half an hour. Strain. Dose: a dessertspoonful to a wineglassful, according to age, three or four times daily. Comfrey makes an excellent cough medicine.

Chamomile, Bran or Linseed Poultices to the chest are also most effective. So are the popular mentholated ointments.

When a child has a coughing spasm raise his left arm high above his head for a moment or so.

For dry, hard and painful coughs try the following:

Fluid extract of Boneset	½ ounce
Tincture of Spongia	½ ounce
Tincture of Ipecacuanha	5 drops

Take five to ten drops in a little warm water four to six times daily. This preparation will give better results if obtained from a homoeopathic chemist, using the same ingredients and quantities of the mother tincture. (see also the advice given under Onion, Whooping Cough, Bronchitis and Lung Weakness)

CRAMP

Vervain herb	½ ounce
Scullcap herb	½ ounce
Wild Yam	½ ounce

Simmer slowly in two pints of water in an iron or enamel pot for twenty minutes. Strain. Take a wineglassful before meals. Sweeten if desired.

Biochemic Mag. Phos. 6x is often most effective. Dissolve three tablets in a tablespoonful of hot water and take three times daily. Try Cuprum 12 if Mag. Phos. fails: four pills morning and night. Hot foot baths are helpful. Affected muscles should be well massaged with Compound Tincture of Myrrh.

CROUP

Homoeopathic remedies are probably the best. Obtain Aconitum 3x and Spongia 3x. Take three or four pills of Aconitum 3x before meals, and three or four of Spongia 3x after meals, three times daily; and another dose of Spongia 3x on retiring. As symptoms abate cease the Aconitum and continue with the Spongia until well. Spinal packs are useful (See Bathing). When the homoeopathic medicines are not available Mag. Phos. 6x may be given: three tablets in hot water three or four times daily. In cases where there is no response professional aid should be obtained, as the cause may be such that expert diagnosis is necessary.

CYSTS

Cysts or wens will often yield to homoeopathic Apis and

Iodine. Take three pills of Apis 30 on rising and a similar dose of Iodine 30 on retiring for about three weeks. Obstinate cysts call for professional attention, preferably homoeopathic or herbal.

DAMIANA

An excellent tonic to the entire system and to the generative organism in particular. Dose: half a teaspoonful of the fluid extract in a little hot water before meals. The homoeopathic fresh plant tincture of Turnera (Damiana) is better, the dose for this being five drops in water before meals. Good for sexual weakness and neurasthenia.

DANDELION

The dried, roasted root of the Dandelion makes excellent coffee, and is beneficial to the liver. It is quite a pleasant beverage. Obtainable from health food stores and herb vendors.

Dandelion leaves added to salads improve the appetite and purify the blood. As a medicine for stomach, liver and bowels simmer an ounce of the sliced roots in a pint of water for fifteen minutes. Strain. Dose: a wineglassful before meals. Flavour with Liquorice if desired.

DANDRUFF

Dandruff points to toxic blood and poor scalp circulation. By building up the system with sane Diet, Bathing, Breathing and Exercise, dandruff should disappear. If the hair is thin, brittle or falling out, see the advice given under **Hair**.

The head should be washed at least once weekly. After drying massage into the scalp oil of Rosemary, or oil of Eucalyptus. Rosemary is pleasant, and the odour of Eucalyptus soon passes. Any hair that comes away when massaging the scalp is dead, and has to come out in any case. By improving circulation in the scalp new hair will grow and dandruff will be eliminated. The writer had a case of neurasthenia in which the patient was totally bald. He was only twenty-two years of age. By means of wise living and natural treatment his general health was restored, and he grew a fine head of glossy hair! A hair specialist had told him that his hair roots were dead, and that he would be bald for life. So much for scientific experts!

Unfortunately, many shampoos are harmful. The best way to wash the scalp is to use M'Clinton's Soap. Failing that, Slippery Elm Soap. Wash the head vigorously, and well rinse out the Soap before drying and using the oil.

One writer advises a mixture of equal parts of distilled extract of Witch Hazel and Eau-de-Cologne. This should be quite satisfactory, but we have had no experience with the mixture. It could be tried instead of one of the oils, if preferred.

'DEAD FINGERS'

When the fingers 'go to sleep', or there is numbness or tingling, there is probably some obstruction in the tissues of the neck and shoulders interfering with nerve supply and circulation. Deep massage of the neck and shoulders is always helpful. If this is not satisfactory visit a good osteopath who will soon correct the trouble. (See also **Neuritis**.)

DEAFNESS, DUE TO CHILL, WAX IN THE EAR

Take the medicine advised for colds, or some hot Composition Powder. Have a really hot foot-bath. As a rule, deafness due to a cold will be eliminated by this method. Deafness due to defects of the auditory mechanism should receive expert attention. Never dabble in so-called cures. What we advise here is for dullness of hearing due solely to a chill, catarrh and resultant deafness. It is the catarrh we are treating.

Wax in the ear can be removed by extracting it with soft tissue wound round the head of a lady's hair pin. Don't prod too deeply. In some cases a few drops of warm Olive or Verbascum oil dropped into the ear will soften the wax and it will come away. Massage round the ear and temple with warm Olive oil. In stubborn cases get an experienced person to syringe the ear. It is not wise to attempt this oneself.

DEBILITY

Treat as for **Anaemia**. Build up the system by means of Breathing exercises, Friction baths and sensible Dieting. Also, remember the vital importance of the right mental attitude to life. Read up the remarks given under **Psychology** and **Spiritual Aid**.

Homoeopathic Arnica 30 is a fine remedy for general debility. Arsenic Alb. 30 also is helpful in some cases. When the heart is weak try Jacaranda 30. If the breathing is sluggish, Rumex Crispus 30 may be the remedy, or Natrum Mur. 30. Arnica may always be tried. To select other remedies look up what is said concerning them in a homoeopathic repertory. The dose for any of the remedies is three or four pills on the tongue morning and night for two or three weeks. To our certain knowledge the application of high frequency (Violet ray) to the head and spine every other day for three weeks has given vitality, restored functional tone and caused many unpleasant symptoms to depart.

DEPRESSION

Sufferers should read what is said on **Psychology** and **Spiritual Aid**. However, the body may be affecting the mind as much as the mind is troubling the body; so build up the general health with Exercise, Breathing and Bathing (Friction Baths, etc.) Live and feed wisely. Medicine as advised for **Neurasthenia** will help if the sufferer is "nervy". There are several fine homoeopathic remedies for depression, and the one which we regard as being the best is Cadmium Sulph. Take four pills in the 200th potency on rising, and a similar dose on retiring — just the two doses. Note the results. May be repeated in a week or so if necessary. Cadmium Sulph. is also an outstanding remedy for influenza, and that complaint is always associated with depression. Two other good remedies are Mezereum 200 and Plumbum 200. Take as for Cadmium Sulph. They may be tried, one at a time, if Cadmium Sulph. fails.

When troubled with a fit of depression, get busy! Be active. The depression devil flees from activity! A hot-foot bath is helpful.

DIARRHOEA

It is unwise to suppress diarrhoea with strong astringent medicines. Diarrhoea means that the bowels are toxic, and that nature is throwing off waste matter. To stop this process by violent means is a mistake.

A reliable homoeopathic medicine which can be taken, and which helps remove the cause (it is not suppressive) is Podophyllum 3. Take three or four pills every three hours.

Additionally, two drops of distilled extract of Witch Hazel in a small wine glass of cold water may be sipped after meals.

If the diarrhoea persists take the following:

Fluid extract of Bayberry	1 ounce
Fluid extract of Raspberry leaves	2 ounces

Dose: Half to one teaspoonful in a little tepid water three times daily. Dysentery may also respond to this remedy, but in these cases it is wise to seek professional help.

An old country remedy was to heat a clean poker red-hot, and then to place the heated end into a tumbler of cold milk, keeping it there for about fifteen seconds. The milk was then taken slowly. This is well worth trying, and it certainly does act very well in some cases. It is not a superstition. Probably the milk becomes charged with iron vibrations (force) and the milk becomes a biochemic potency of iron. Iron in biochemic form is one of the cures for diarrhoea.

DIET

Do we live to eat, or eat to live? Surely the latter is the object; yet with so many people the idea is to eat solely for pleasure. As the Bible says of such: 'Their god is in their bellies'.

Food should be natural, as provided by nature. Faked foods with chemical additions are not fit for pigs let alone humans. How the system manages to deal with such concoctions is one of the wonders of the day in which we live. The body is designed to deal with organic substances only, yet it is called upon to digest and assimilate vast quantities of lime (as added, for example, to our loaf of white bread), soda, magnesium and small quantities of other inorganic items. Of course they cannot be assimilated. All they do is to place stresses on the digestive and eliminative organs, clog the system, harden the arteries and cause a number of diseases.

The food makes the blood, and the blood is the life of all animal organisms. We hear of the hardy pioneers in new countries, and the reason why they are hardy (were hardy is more correct, as most pioneering is a thing of the past as far as the earth is concerned) is because they had to feed on the natural produce of the virgin soil in new lands; soil that had not been poisoned with chemicals. The plants they fed upon were rich in 'organized' minerals, natural sugars and vitamins. Thus, they became healthy and strong.

HOW TO EAT

First let us deal with the function of eating, for *how* we eat is very important. Then we can discuss what we should eat.

The process of digestion begins in the mouth. By chewing, the saliva is mixed with the food and made ready for the stomach to receive it for the next step in the digestive process. The mouth is the house of preparation. The saliva is a highly organised bio-chemical liquid, and unless it is mixed with the food by the action of mastication, very little good will result from the food eaten. The saliva helps to convert starches into sugar, and unless this is done in the mouth the food will enter the stomach unprepared for the next processing. There will be fermentation and acidity. The poorly prepared and somewhat toxic substance will then pass into the duodenum and intestines, mixed with juices supplied by the liver and other organs. But it is not in the state it should be, and there is general upset in the bowels. This leads to constipation, diarrhoea, auto-toxaemia, acidity, rheumatism, depression, nerviness and diseases too numerous to mention; for it is well known that most diseases have their origin in toxic bowels.

Even poor food will do some good if thoroughly masticated. Small meals, when the food is thoroughly chewed up, will noruish the body. Large meals, eaten quickly, will give the system the devil's own job to clear out the resultant toxins, and actual nourishment will be small. Of course, a biologically strong person, with vigorous organs, will deal with the mess that has been eaten far better than a weakly soul. Anyway, thorough mastication will make the strong stronger, and give more vitality to the weak. We have known feeble, thin and anaemic people put on weight and increase their vital energy by doing nothing more than spend more time over meals, and chew thoroughly all their food. Food should be liquefied in the mouth before swallowing. So, no matter what you eat, do CHEW IT! The best of healthy food will do little good unless it is masticated. Remember this, or the advice that follows will not be of much value.

WHEN TO EAT

Eat when you are hungry, and not because it is a set meal time. We agree that regularity with meals is important; but if not hungry at meal time, do not eat. The system cannot digest food that is not wanted.

It is a mistake to force food upon invalids and sick people when even the sight of it causes nausea. Any food eaten in such circumstances cannot do any good, but places added strain on the weakened organs. Animals are guided by instinct, and they will not eat when they are ill. Civilization, so-called, has killed natural instinct in many respects; although sick people still reject food unless it is forced upon them. Actually, the energy derived from food is small compared with that due to the intake of oxygen. One may do without food for weeks, without water for days; but when it comes to air life flickers out in a minute or so without the act of respiration. So air is more important than food.

It is not our object to encourage food fadding and fussing over meals. Many who are faddy about food are poor specimens of health, for their over-attention to what they eat makes them introspective, and that state of mind breeds disease. As Jesus of Nazareth implied: what comes out of the mouth is more important than what goes into it. One can be poisoned more by thoughts put into words that come out of the mouth than by what is taken internally. Evil speaking poisons the mind and body, and those that listen; while at least the system can deal with the intake of wrong food up to a point. However, wise feeding is not fadding. Let us be reasonable! And, as St. Paul said, 'Let your moderation be known —.'

Never eat when very tired, distressed, upset or angry. If you do you will invite an attack of indigestion.

Owing to the mistaken idea that all energy comes from food, and also because of a false and excessive appetite, most of us eat far too much, and have too many meals. We have known people eat an enormous breakfast consisting of clogging foods, have a snack about 11 a.m., indulge in a hearty lunch, followed by tea in the afternoon. Then, a dinner of sufficient quantity to supply nourishment for twenty-four hours. Later on a big supper to complete the list. Then, wonder of wonders, some get up in the middle of the night and dash to the pantry to keep up their strength! The mental and bodily energy of such people is devoted almost entirely to the digestion and elimination of food.

An animal in the wilds has one good meal daily, and takes a rest after feeding. This is a good example to human beings; after a heavy meal take a rest and relax, if it is at all possible — even if only for a few minutes. Weakly folk should always rest after dinner.

Eating is very much a habit. One can be amply nourished by taking one large meal a day, and one or two smaller meals. The largest meal should be taken in the evening when this is possible. A big breakfast is not good. It is mainly before mid-day that the body eliminates waste matter, and builds up later in the day; so it is more in accord with nature to feed lightly before noon. Late suppers do not suit most people, and much insomnia is caused by eating late. On the other hand there are many sufferers from insomnia who benefit from a cup of hot milk or other food-beverage before retiring. We all differ, and there is no set law for everybody.

WHAT TO EAT

There are people who go from one natural healer to another seeking new curative diets. Such rarely get well, for they are too concerned with themselves. The writer got into a spot of trouble on one occasion by refusing to give a new diet to a woman who had been to a number of practitioners and received a different diet sheet from each of them. She was a neurotic, and was far too concerned with foods and fancies. An attempt was made to treat her psychologically, but she was upset and angry, and reported the writer to his Professional Association for refusing to pander to her wishes.

Always remember that real hunger is present only when the mouth waters, which shows that there is ample saliva ready for the first stage of digestion. It is unwise to eat with a dry, parched mouth. Sauces and condiments tend to produce a false hunger; most of these should be avoided, or taken in strict moderation. We shall deal with this subject later.

It does not follow that the suggestions made in these pages will suit everybody. Some can tackle salads and raw food;

others cannot. It is wrong to insist, as some practitioners do, that everybody *must* eat raw food. It is useless trying to eat what one canot digest, and also to partake of some special healing food that is very distasteful. Trying to eat what one really does not like means that the digestive system is not stimulated by the mind to receive such food, and food taken under protest cannot achieve much good no matter how valuable it is. To desire and like food means that it is half digested before it enters the mouth, for the mental attitude stimulates the digestive secretions.

Of course we have to guard against perverted appetites, such as a craving for alcohol and sweets. But there are pleasing substitutes for such things. It is for the reader to select from the hints given what he or she likes, and follow the advice as far as reasonably possible. Every effort in the right direction is a help.

1. Raw food is usually easily digested if it is well masticated, so have at least one salad daily, dressed with Olive, nut or sunflower seed oil and Lemon juice. Salads may consist of any fresh vegetables in season, and the fresher they are the better. Shredded cabbage, Balm, Thyme, Sage, etc., may be added to any salad. Also, items which may be included in salads to the advantage of the general health are Dandelion leaves, rose petals, nasturtium leaves and seeds, Violet leaves, Clover flowers, etc. The appearance of a salad can be made very tempting by arranging these items nicely on the dish. Many people cannot digest Radishes and cucumber. Before discarding such foods try eating them with their tops and rinds. That is, eat the Radish tops with the roots and the peel on the cucumber. Nature has so arranged the chemistry of these vegetables that items in the tops and rinds help the digestion. Fruits such as apples, dates, raisins and oranges may also be added to salads. Also, for those who can digest them, ground nuts. With the salad, potatoes, boiled or baked in their jackets, may be taken in moderation. The only condiments added, apart from Lemon juice (no Vinegar) should be best Cayenne (red) pepper, genuine black pepper and Sea Salt (from chemists). Avoid white pepper and ordinary Salt. Those with irritable stomachs should avoid condiments. Pure food, properly grown, supplies all the mineral salts necessary. Finely cut, or pulverized herbs may

also be sprinkled over both salads and cooked meals. Such prepared herbs can be obtained from health food stores. Cheese or meat may be taken with salads. For those with weak digestions the cheese should be either cottage cheese, lactic cheese or ordinary cheese that has been flaked, spread out on a dish and allowed to dry for a few hours. Meats should be mutton, poultry or white fish for preference.

2. Sufferers from some disorders require special diets, and must keep to foods they have been advised to eat. Diabetics are an example. These hints are suitable for most people. Never be afraid of good food, for fear of food means that you will be unable to digest it.

3. Have fresh fruit as available. Apples may be sliced or grated, and added to salads. Also oranges, dates, sultanas, etc.

4. Fresh eggs, in moderation, are good for most people. They should be either scrambled or lightly boiled. Fried eggs are not ideal, but there is no reason why you should not have a fried egg sometimes if your stomach can digest it. There are a few people who cannot tolerate eggs in any form, and such should eliminate them from their meals.

5. Genuine, compost-grown wholemeal bread should replace white (See **Bread**). Bread is better eaten stale. Stout people would be better for taking Swedish Rye Biscuits in place of bread. Those who, by reason of inflamed membranes or duodenal ulceration, cannot take Bran should avoid wholemeal bread, as the Bran will irritate. Until well, such should have bread free from Bran, but containing the wheat germ. 'Hovis' is an example.

6. Most people would be better for a laxative breakfast, whether habitually constipated or not. (See **Constipation**.)

7. A little wheat germ such as 'Bemax' or 'Froment' sprinkled over any meal will benefit the brain and nerves. These foods are rich in the B vitamins and certain minerals.

8. Yeast foods are excellent for the nerves and appetite taken as beverages, spreads or added to gravy. They will often restore a jaded appetite.

9. White sugar is a curse. All tests by food scientists show that it is decidedly harmful, not only to the teeth but to the constitution generally. Use common moist brown sugar; or, better still, replace by pure, natural Honey — even for sweetening beverages.

10. Beverages are better taken a few minutes before feeding,

and this applies especially to warm drinks. Dandelion coffee is very good for the stomach, liver and blood. Diluted fruit juices, or vegetable juices, are fine. But be sure to use fresh juice, or juice guaranteed to be free from chemical preservatives. All bottled juice is to be regarded with suspicion. Read the label, and if it says that a certain percentage, no matter how minute of any chemical has been added, then that juice is not ideal, and may even harm some constitutions.

11. Weakly people and those with delicate digestions will derive much help from Slippery Elm food (from chemists and health food stores). A cup of this food is a meal in itself when there is no desire for more food.

12. Always be happy at the meal table. Happineşs aids digestion.

WHAT NOT TO EAT

1. Avoid shell fish, eels, game, goose, duck and the flesh of the pig. At least do this as far as is reaonably possible. These fish and animals are scavengers, and their flesh is not by any means ideal as food for humans. The ancient laws given by Moses prohibited such foods; and not without good, scientific reasons. These laws are perfect for flesh-eaters.

2. Vegetarians should not eat large quantities of starch in an effort to replace meat. The soya bean is a very fine food. Peas, beans and lentils also replace meat. It is not the purpose of the writer to cater for vegetarians only, or to argue on the subject. The idea is to present sensible rules for both meat eaters and vegetarians.

3. Be moderate with all fried foods. Very little pastry. Both cake and pastry should be made with fine wholemeal flour. Those with weak digestions and faulty livers should avoid fried foods entirely.

4. Avoid condiments except for small quantities of finely cut or powdered herbs, genuine Red or Black Pepper and a very little Sea Salt. No Vinegar (unless advised as a medicine — see Apple Cider Vinegar). Replace Vinegar with pure Lemon juice.

5. Avoid sauces. If you must have sauce use it sparingly.

6. Avoid strong tea and coffee. Both are harmful stimulants when taken to excess. Weak tea is in order, and it should be sweetened with Honey or moist brown sugar. Small cups of hot black coffee may be taken to tone the stomach (as a

medicine) before heavy meals in some cases; but only for short periods.

7. Avoid 'the miseries' at the meal table. A happy state of mind, and pleasant conversation, will aid digestion.

8. Do not boil or cook in Aluminium utensils (See **Aluminium**).

9. It is wise to make any changes in the diet gradually.

10. Be very moderate with alcohol, especially spirits. Many are better without any. However, a little good wine before or after meals acts as a stomach tonic to many. All pseudo-religious 'kill-joys' should remember that St. Paul told Timothy to 'take a little wine for his stomach's sake'. Weakly folk may derive benefit from an occasional glass of stout.

11. The too frequent use of cooked animal fats upsets the liver and causes circulatory trouble. Many cases of blood clot (Thrombosis) would never have taken place if the sufferer had taken less animal fat. For cooking purposes use Olive, sunflower or maize oil. Nut oils are also permissible. Shun animal fats and keep your arteries young.

12. Do not get a craze for Vitamins. We all need Vitamins, and all natural foods are rich in these elements. Too many synthetic Vitamins may not be advisable, and far too many preparations in the chemists contain inorganic minerals as well as Vitamins. Take Vitamins as provided by nature. Shun all synthetic, man-made food substitutes.

THE DAILY FOOD

Here is an example of health meals for one day which should meet the requirements of the average person.

Breakfast Cereal, such as Shredded Wheat, or uncooked rolled Oats, with a little 'All-Bran' if constipated. Prunes. Moisten the cereal with prune juice. The prunes should be soaked overnight in some water to which half a small teaspoonful of Molasses has been added. Prunes and Agar-Agar are ideal if constipated; otherwise use dates, figs, raisins, etc. A cup of weak tea or Dandelion Coffee may be taken before or after the meal; or a glass of fruit or vegetable juice.

Lunch Have either a good salad consisting of items suggested in the hints given, or a cooked meal consisting of Potatoes baked or boiled in their jackets, conservatively cooked or steamed vegetables, with cheese or one of the flesh foods advised. Whether a salad or a cooked meal is eaten, it may be preceded by a bowl of good vegetable soup, if desired.

Beverages, as suggested in these hints, may be taken a few minutes before or after eating. Those with weak digestions may benefit by drinking at least fifteen minutes before feeding. If desired lunch may be followed by fruit or a sweet made from natural, wholesome ingredients.

Tea A cup of weak tea, Dandelion Coffee or fruit juice. A wholemeal biscuit if desired.

Dinner Vegetable stew followed by wholemeal bread and butter pudding. Or exactly the same as for lunch. Wise people will have two salads most days, but if you have a cooked meal for lunch have a salad for dinner; or vice versa.

Another suggestion for lunch or dinner: scrambled eggs on wholemeal toast; or, lightly boiled eggs with wholemeal or crispbread.

Supper Not advisable, but some people sleep better if they have a cup of warm milk with half a teaspoonful of plain extract of malt added; or a cup of Slippery Elm food. A glass of stout for those who wish.

CURATIVE PROPERTIES OF SOME FOODS

Apples Excellent for the brain and nerves. Purify the blood and clean the teeth. They are cooling in fevers. 'An apple a day keeps the doctor away', is good sense up to a point. Apples are good for those suffering from shingles. Invalids may have them cooked, but without sugar — use Honey.

Artichokes: Good for the nerves and heart.

Asparagus: There is ample proof that this is a help in cases of weak heart. Tones arteries and kidneys.

Bananas: Eat only when ripe. Good for the thin, especially when baked.

Barley Water: When made from pot barley this is helpful in cases of inflamed urinary organs. Soothing and healing.

Blackberries: Valuable in anaemia, digestive trouble and bowel weakness.

Carrots: Good for the nerves, digestive organs, kidneys and the sight. Of some value in asthma.

Celery: Helpful to the nervous system and cleansing to the blood. A good food for neurasthenia and rheumatism.

Currants: Some value as blood cleansers.

Dandelion Leaves: Added to salads they activate the liver and help to purify the blood. Have digestive properties.

Dates: Supply energy and are very easily digested. Better than sweets from the shops.

Figs: Very good blood purifiers. Have laxative properties, especially black Spanish figs. (See also **Figs** as discussed elsewhere).

Grapes: A mineral-rich food. Easily digested and very good for invalids, and those with weak digestions. A food for anaemia. Both the blue and green varieties are brimful of tonic and nourishing properties. Grapes are better eaten alone, or with dates.

Lemons: Powerful, natural antiseptics. Make a healing and refreshing beverage for colds, fevers and throat affections. Rich in vitamin C. Vitamin P is also present, and this helps to tone the arteries and capillaries; hence Lemon is good for arterial disease and high blood pressure.

Lettuce: Has some value in nervous weakness. Calming to the brain.

Maize Oil: The system handles this oil without harm resulting to the liver and blood chemistry. Very good for cooking.

Oats: Excellent nerve builders. They suit some people when eaten as rolled Oats, without cooking. Add from a teaspoonful to a dessertspoonful to other breakfast cereals. Should be well masticated. Helpful for acid stomach.

Onions: Antiseptic. Good for colds. Help to prevent auto-toxaemia. Garlic is more powerful.

Oranges: Similar to the Lemon, but not so effective for colds and fevers. Excellent for most people, although oranges do not suit some people who have sluggish livers.

Olive Oil: Excellent for salads. Improves the skin and strengthens the nerves. A little Olive oil, thoroughly emulsified by mixing one or two teaspoonsful with some hot malted milk and very thoroughly shaken up, or prepared in a mechanical mixer, is a wonderful food in cases of nervous exhaustion.

Parsley: A little fresh parsley cut up and sprinkled over salads or cooked meals in an excellent tonic for the kidneys and bladder. Claimed to be helpful in female irregularities.

Pineapples: Very good for feeble digestion. Tough parts should be rejected.

Prunes: Gently laxative. Very good for the liver and blood.

Raisins: Both raisins and sultanas are rich in natural sugar. They are good for the blood, and supply energy.

Runner Beans: A wonderful food for the kidneys and bladder. Aid the heart. See also the special remarks on **Runner Beans** in the text.

Slippery Elm: Slippery Elm food, obtainable from herbal, health food stores and chemists, is one of the very best curative foods for troubles of the digestive organs. It is fine for ulceration, and its influence extends to all organs of the body. Very nourishing.

Strawberries: When fully ripe have some value in anaemia, liver weakness and rheumatism.

Sunflower Seed Oil: Ideal for cooking. It is claimed that it strengthens the sight, tones the arteries and gives energy.

Turnips: Turnip juice is good for stomach and duodenal ulceration. Claimed to be helpful for weak sight.

Water Cress: A blood cleanser. Has some general tonic value.

Water (Soft): Soft water, taken freely, helps to dissolve uric acid, flush the kidneys and cleanse the system of impurities. In some institutions soft water is used as a cure for many disorders due to self-poisoning and morbid material in the system. A tumbler is taken slowly six to twelve times daily, with very little food, for a few days. People with heart trouble are not advised to attempt this, as in these cases an excess of liquid in the system is harmful. The same may apply in some high blood pressure cases. Otherwise, it is a perfectly harmless 'cure' which may be tried at home, with only good resulting. Water is nature's natural beverage. Unfortunately what comes from the tap these days is usually chlorinated, and can cause harm in many instances. It is most difficult in our time to get away from the chemicalisation of foods and beverages.

MIXTURES AND COMBINATIONS

Several kinds of food at one meal can be tackled by those with good digestions; but people who have weak stomachs would do well to avoid too much variety; the weaker the digestion the greater the care that should be taken.

It is helpful not to take two kinds of protein at one meal. For instance, do not have both meat *and* cheese. To a lesser degree the same rule applies to starches. If you have bread do not have Potatoes at the same time. The stomach sufferer is advised not to have three different kinds of food at any one time. He or she can have fruit and protein or fruit and starch; but not starch, fruit and protein together. In severe cases a Mono-Diet is often helpful. That is to say, one kind of food only at any one meal. But this is rather trying and most uninteresting, and applies only to those whose digestive organs are in a very bad condition. Such would do well to go on 'baby foods' in order to give the stomach and other organs a rest, and a chance to build up. Slippery Elm food, Arrowroot and those advertised foods recommended for babies are usually helpful in these cases for a short period of time. When it is sick the stomach needs rest above all things.

Here is a recipe for sufferers from weak stomachs. This will supply all the nourishment, vitamins and minerals needed for some days; but it is not intended to be the sole food over long periods. A week on this food can accomplish much good in many cases. It gives the stomach a partial rest.

To a cup of cold, fresh milk add a teaspoonful of powdered gum Acacia, one of Agar-Agar, and a quarter of a small teaspoonful of powdered Kelp (Bladderwrack). Mix thoroughly. Place this in a cereal bowl and add some clean dates and a *ripe* banana. Use a fork and mash the whole together. Those who like an acid taste may add some mashed ripe apple, or Lemon juice. Apart from the Acacia, Agar-Agar and Kelp the quantity of each ingredient may be varied to one's liking. The dates should be soft, and any hard parts omitted. Eat slowly. May be taken two or three times daily for a week or so, and then eaten for breakfast only. If constipated, prunes may be mashed in with the other ingredients. The prunes may be soaked in the milk overnight and half a teaspoonful of Molasses added.

Those who dislike Kelp may omit this ingredient. Some may like to mix the powders in a little warm milk before adding cold.

DIPHTHERIA

When uncertain about a throat condition, and fever is

present, it is wise to seek professional aid. A helpful and reliable medicine consists of two parts fluid extract of Echinacea and one part Tincture of Myrrh. Give the sufferer two to five drops in a little warm water every two hours. Neat Lemon juice poured into the sufferer's throat in frequent, but quite small quantities has been known to keep a membrane from forming, and has saved life. Many years ago the writer knew a boy whose life was saved by his mother giving Lemon in this manner after the local doctor had given up hope. (See also **Sore Throat**).

DOCTRINE OF SIGNATURES (See Laws of Correspondence)

DROPSY

Lily-of-the Valley	½ ounce
Broom tops	1 ounce
Dandelion root	½ ounce

Simmer gently in two pints of water for fifteen minutes. Strain. Take a tablespoonful to a wineglassful three our four times daily. This is a very good remedy to regulate the water in the system and strengthen the heart and kidneys.

See also the **Runner Bean** treatment.

A homoeopathic method of dealing with dropsy is to take five pills of Apis Mel. 3x before meals, and five of Spartium 1x after meals, three times daily. If the heart is very weak take Strophanthus 1x instead of Apis Mel.

DYSPEPSIA (See Indigestion)

EAR ACHE

With the feet in a bowl of really hot water, press cold cloths to the back of the neck. This often brings instant relief.

Another way is to apply the middle finger-tip to the ear. Hold the finger horizontally, keeping the other fingers and thumb lightly clenched, so that the middle finger-tip enters the ear and makes *light* contact. Then twist the finger to the right, and then to the left, making the circular twisting movements fairly quickly. There is considerable human magnetism in the middle finger, and this operation, continued for a minute or two, has taken away the pain in many instances known to the writer. May be repeated several times at intervals. Naturally one has to have the finger nail short — a finger with a claw instead of a trimmed nail is useless.

A little warm Verbascum oil in the ear will be helpful when other means fail. Homoeopathic Aconitum 3x and Pulsatilla 3x are useful medicines. We have known them act very quickly. Take four pills of Aconitum 3x and about fifteen minutes later four of Pulsatilla 3x. If the pain does not go repeat in an hour's time. Other remedies more suitable in some cases, and taken in the same manner, are Mercurius 8x and Apil Mel. 3x.

Hot salt bags are very effective (see under **Salt**). It is wise to obtain professional aid in removing hard wax from the ear. Verbascum oil in the ear occasionally will soften wax and render its removal an easier operation. When this oil is not available use warm Olive oil.

EARTH AND CLAY

Some native peoples, including the American Indians, lay great stress on earth treatment. As one Indian Chief said: 'Great Spirit, him strong in the tress and powerful in the air; but him mighty powerful down there!' Meaning, that the healing power was strong in leaves and herbs, powerful in the air (Breathing), but very powerful indeed in the earth. The custom is to bury sufferers from all manner of diseases in the earth up to their necks, leave them there for some hours, and then remove them. Observers tell us that the astonishing thing is that many are cured. The reason probably is that the body draws unto itself the healing minerals and something of the earth's magnetism. Do we not call our planet 'mother earth'? This earth-mother supplies us with our food in the plant kingdom, and there is no reason why direct and full contact with her cannot supply energy and other essentials. The sand of the sea is likewise effective. A baby girl of nine months had rheumatic fever, which was followed by paralysis. All medical treatment failed. Then, at the age of five, she was buried in sea sand up to her shoulders for an hour every day. After fourteen days she recovered and walked. This little girl had treatment from the writer for the effects of an accident when she was fifty-six! Celebrated doctors and the wise men may laugh; but we are interested in results and not so much in 'the wisdom of this world'. 'The world, by wisdom, knew not God'. No doubt to be steeped in worldly wisdom can close the mind to instinct and common sense. We are all for knowledge, but have no time for professionalism and so-called science when they are little better than stupidity. Scientific snobbery is a curse of the age.

In natural treatment institutes clean clay is employed as packs and compresses for feverish conditions, sprains and injuries. Sore and stiff joints will yield to its influence. Moist clay applied as an ointment to the anus is good for piles.

To make a clay pack dig for the cleanest clay to be found. Get out as much grit and stone as possible, mix with a little cold water and apply as a thick paste on linen to any painful joint, sore or injury. It is better not to apply when the skin is broken unless one can be absolutely certain that the clay is free from every kind of contamination – which is rarely possible. A large compress over the abdomen, and kept on all night, will do much to clear up all abdominal complains and some female disorders. It can be tried when the more orthodox methods fail. The results are often amazing!

Ladies use clay for beauty treatments, and this happens to be one of the few sensible applications that can be made to the face.

Jesus made clay ointment to anoint the eyes of a blind man to restore his sight. We may be sure that the clay was necessary or he would not have used it. From this we gather that faith is not enough for all cures as some would have us believe. 'Faith without works is dead!' Yes, an ointment made by moistening clean clay can do more to heal sores and injuries than many expensive ointments. Also, it is not suppressive.

ECHINACEA

This plant is a most valuable cleanser of the blood. It also acts on the gall bladder and prostate gland, giving tone to both these organs. In our opinion it is superior to any of the modern drugs as an antiseptic and purifier of the system. The dose is half a teaspoonful of the fluid extract in hot water before meals. Useful for all blood and skin diseases, congested gall bladder and enlarged prostate gland. For those who prefer to take it homoeopathically the dose is four or five pills of the 3x potency three times daily. Even better results may follow taking the 30th potency morning and night for two or three weeks.

ECZEMA

The herbal recipe given for **Auto-toxaemia** is very good for eczema and other skin disorders. The fluid extract of Burdock has been known to clear up the trouble if taken for some time: half a teaspoonful in half a cup of hot water before or after meals, three times daily.

The only soaps used should be M'Clinton's or Slippery Elm. In severe cases Rumex ointment (supplied by homoeopathic chemists) may be smeared over the irritable patches twice daily. There are several good homoeopathic medicines which can be taken internally, if the sufferer prefers to use homoeopathy instead of herbs. It is wasteful to take both at the same time. Four pills of Arsen. Alb. 6 and four of Rhus Tox. 3, taken alternately every three or four hours have proved most effective in some cases. Other good remedies are: Drosera 3, Hydrocotyle 3, Graphites 6 and Euphorbium 3. Read up these remedies in a homoeopathic repertory and select the one that seems to cover your particular symptoms.

For local bathing. Two tablespoonsful of Epsom salts to two pints of warm water. Sponge the areas twice daily.

ELDER FLOWERS

A fine ancient remedy for colds, fevers, coughs and bronchitis. Has cleared asthma when expensive treatment has failed. Also of much value to the nervous system. Simmer an ounce of the flowers in a pint of water, using an iron or enamel pot, for fifteen minutes. Keep the lid on and simmer very gently. Strain. Dose: a dessertspoonful to a wineglassful, according to age, three or four times daily. Elder flowers combined with an equal part of Peppermint herb, prepared as above, with an eggspoonful of Composition Powder added, will make short work of most colds and is good for influenza. Sambucus Nig. (Elder) in the 3rd or 30th homoeopathic potency, is more powerfully acting in many cases. Take four or five pills of the 3rd potency three or four times daily, or the 30th morning and night only. Sambucus Nig. in potency is a fine remedy for asthma.

ELECAMPANE

Another old remedy worthy of praise for coughs. Prepare and take as for Elder Flower medicine. The homoeopathic name is Inula, and in the 30th potency it is very effective for fibrositis. A dose of four or five pills morning and night.

EMACIATION

Treat as for Anaemia. The cause is usually wrong food eaten too quickly. Go by the hints given under Diet, and also indulge in Breathing exercises and Friction baths. Stop worrying.

EMERGENCIES (See Camphor, Cayenne and Breathing)

EMETICS

Many herbalists regard the administration of an emetic as being a first essential step in the treatment of many ailments due to toxaemia, and especially for stomach, liver and bowel disorders. Attacks of asthma can often be aborted by taking an emetic and during an attack prompt relief is obtained.

A very efficient emetic consists of one or two teaspoonsful of the Acid Tincture of Lobelia and five to ten drops of Tincture of Capsicum in about three quarters of a tumbler of tepid water. The dose for children should be less according to age. This is not recommended for the very young unless given under professional supervision.

Another reliable emetic is a teaspoonful of English Mustard in a tumbler of warm water. If necessary this may be repeated two or three times at ten minute intervals.

Ipecacuanha Wine had been used as an emetic for a very long time. The dose ranges from about ten drops to six teaspoonsful, according to age. The smaller doses are good for coughs, but even the young need one to three teaspoonsful in order to induce vomiting.

Drinking a large quantity of tepid water will sometimes cause vomiting.

Many cases of indigestion, biliousness and general morbidness can be banished very quickly by taking an emetic. In the animal world the first thing a sick creature does is to make itself vomit. We can learn a great deal by observing the instinctive habits of animals.

EMOTIONS

Hate, envy, anger, jealousy and all the ugly, vicious brood of evil emotions poison the brain and blood more than all the wrong feeding. To indulge in these emotions for only a few moments upsets the brain, nerves and circulation. They are injurious to the heart, mar the complexion and keep one in the mire. They prepare the way for all manner of both mental and physical disease. On the other hand, the emotions of joy, happiness and good-will bring more health and peace of mind and body to the giver than they do to the receiver. They brighten the mind, improve the circulation and are a tonic to all the organic processes. Hate, for example, will retard digestion and poison the food; love will aid digestion and improve nutrition. See also **Psychology, Spiritual Aid, Anger.** Many a disease has been made worse because the sufferer bore ill-will to somebody, or was resentful about something; many a disorder has been cleared up, when medicine has failed, by a change of heart and mind on the part of the sufferer.

EPSOM SALTS

The frequent use of large doses of Epsom Salts as a purgative weakens the bowels. See under **Constipation** for more suitable remedies. However, there are cases of indigestion, acidity and rheumatism that may be helped by taking a mere pinch of these salts in a small tumbler of hot water morning and night, first and last thing. The small dose is very unlike the larger one — one might say that the small is a low potency homoeopathic medicine.

The chief use for Epsom Salts is in the bath. Obtain the cheap Epsom from the chemists; as used for cattle. Add a good double handful, more or less, to an ordinary bath of hot water. When in the bath rub the body all over for a minute or two with the wet hands. The action is over quickly. Do not use Soap for these baths. The salts draw acids and toxins through the skin. Rheumatic sufferers will derive benefit from such a bath taken once or twice weekly. Five minutes in the bath are ample.

ERYNGO

This plant is usually known as Seaholly. It has a wide range of action, and is given for coughs, kidney and bladder weakness, dropsy, liver and spleen congestion and as a general tonic. Preparation and doses as for **Elder flowers**. This harmless remedy may be tried by all sufferers from the complaints mentioned, with most beneficial results.

ERYSIPELAS

A good herbal medicine is the one advised for **Auto-Toxaemia**. Rhus Tox. 3x has cured many cases; four pills three times daily. Tablets of Hepar Sulph. 3x have also been effective. Other homoeopathic remedies are: Anarcardium Occ., Crotalus Hor., Gelsemium, Clematis, Kali Chloride and Silica. Sufferers are urged not to experiment, but to visit a reliable homoeopathic or herbal practitioner.

EUCALYPTUS

Oil of Eucalyptus is one of the finest antiseptics provided by the vegetable kingdom. For those who are afraid of germs it is equal to anything the chemists can create as a germ killer, and far less harmful.

The oil, inhaled, is refreshing and stimulating. In colds and catarrh it soothes the respiratory passages and helps to free them from obstruction. Fairly frequent inhalation helps to free the lungs, and gives relief in bronchitis, fevers and throat disorders.

As a medicine one or two drops on brown sugar or Honey may be taken two or three times daily to speed up cure in such conditions. The oil may also be rubbed into the chest and back. Another method in respiratory disorders is to drop some oil onto a piece of blotting paper and place it next to the chest beneath a garment. The fumes will rise and be inhaled gradually.

A tea made from the leaves of the Eucalyptus tree is most useful in all types of fever, septic conditions and catarrh. Place one ounce of the leaves in a pint of hot water in a jug. Cover, and allow to stand for half an hour. Strain. Dose: a wineglassful every three or four hours. Or, employ the fluid extract, when the dose is half a small teaspoonful in warm water. The tea made from the leaves is also healing and cleaning when applied to ulcers as a compress.

Another tree of the same family, Eucalyptus Citriodora, is sweetly scented, and is most pleasant to inhale for colds and catarrh.

EUPHORBIUM

This is a drastic purgative, and we do not advise its use in material doses. Even one drop will purge the bowels. Homoeopathically it becomes a wonderful medicine with an exceptionally wide range of action. It has a tonic and normalising effect on the mucous membranes, veins, capillaries, duodenum, intestines, bones, fibrous tissue, skin, ovaries, pituitary gland, suprarenal glands, Thyroid, parathyroids and the haemoglobin. A remedy having an action on so many organs and endocrine glands is very unusual, although Fucus (Bladderwrack) taken homoeopathically is another example. Euphorbium 6, four pills morning and night, may be taken for disorders associated with any of the organs mentioned when other treatments fail to produce results. But, in our opinion, this is one of those remedies which is better prescribed by a skilled practitioner. Given correctly it is a wonderful medicine. In the case of Euphorbium a homoeopathic repertory is not of great value as most of the findings respecting its action have been made by means of radiesthesia.

EVENING PRIMROSE

A tea made from the Evening Primrose has a very profound action in gastro-intestinal disorders of a functional origin. It seems to act on the organs of digestion and assimilation via the mind; hence, it will often produce results in sensitive, nervy people, and those upset by worry and anxiety. Those suffering from any kind of digestive or bowel trouble who cannot find the right medicine, and who have upsetting problems on their minds, can try this harmless medicine. Only good can result. Simmer an ounce of the leaves in a pint of water for fifteen minutes. Strain. Take a tablespoonful before meals.

EXERCISE

Life is movement! The more life there is in a person the more active he is. It is in the nature of things that movement is essential to living, and the circulation of the blood and the functional tone of all bodily organs are improved by exercise. The way to strengthen a muscle is to use it, and the same applies to the organs of the body. However, vigorous exercise should never be undertaken by weakly people. For such, exercise is necessary (unless confined to bed or an invalid chair) but it must be gentle.

A great rule for all is never to exercise to the extent of feeling fatigued. Up to a certain point exercise will do good; after that point has been reached, harm may result.

For many people, walking is one of the best exercises; not just strolling along, but walking briskly, with the head high, the chin in, the abdomen in and the chest wall held out. If you keep the chin and abdomen in, and the shoulders back and down, you will have assumed the best posture. (See **Posture**). Breathing exercises can be indulged in while taking a walk (See **Breathing**). Walking has a stimulating effect on all functional activity in the organism. In these mechanical days many have almost forgotten how to walk, and a tensed-up, nervy and sorry crowd we are! Always enjoy your walk, and it will do you more good.

If you are fit enough, take a run sometimes. Most games are good forms of exercise: horse riding, skipping, football, cricket, tennis, etc. Select your games according to your abilities.

Weight-lifting, with due caution, can be a very health-giving exercise. Wrestling and boxing are good for those capable of entering such sports.

For the sedentary worker, and the weakly person who wants to build up his body, we place walking and breathing first. Here are a few simple exercises that can do good to all, except those who are bed-ridden — or almost!

1. Stretching. Yes, stretching is an exercise, and all stretching should be done before and after other exercises. Stretching is good for the spine, and a strong spine does much to keep the body vigorous. All animals stretch. Watch them. Observe the cat cling to the tree trunk with his front claws and stretch.

Clasp the hands, palms upward, above the head and stretch up as much as possible. Relax, and do it six to twelve times. Stretch out each limb separately, several times; even stretch the fingers.

2. Stand erect, chin in, chest out, and raise the hands over the head. Bend down and try to touch the toes. Bring the arms up, and repeat several times. Do not bend the knees.

3. Arms over the head. Turn to the right, making the movement from the hips, and bend over and downwards as far as you can. Repeat from the left side. Do this several times.

4. Hold the arms out from the sides, shoulder high. Keep the hands limp. Stand erect and, swinging the trunk from the hips, throw the arms vigorously first to one side and then to the other from six to twelve times.

5. Stand or sit erectly. Stretch the head backwards as far as possible; then bring it forwards allowing the chin to *fall* on the chest. Then place the clasped hands behind the neck and press the head forwards. It may hurt somewhat, and this shows just how much this neck stretch is needed. Repeat several times.

6. From the same position turn the head to the right as far as possible, but *keep the chin in.* Then to the left. Repeat several times. The neck contains several organs and is a very congested part of the anatomy. Head and neck bending and twisting will do much to improve the circulation in this area, free impinged nerves and aid the system generally. When performing this exercise endeavour to get the chin over each shoulder without tilting the head.

These few exercises are enough for the average person. The weakly can do what they can manage without fatigue or discomfort, and each movement may be done less frequently. Even when in bed stretching can be managed, and one may bend forwards, try to touch the toes, and also bring the feet up over the head, balancing the body with the elbows. The latter movements should be tried only a few times at first until the abdominal muscles have been strengthened.

Remember to indulge in some breathing exercises before

and after physical movements. Even five minutes a day devoted to exercise will pay rich dividends in health. Master your body; do not allow it to master your mind.

EXHAUSTION

See **Collapse.** Homoeopathic Acid Phos. 1x is also very good for exhaustion. Take three or four drops in an egg cup of cold water before meals.

EYEBRIGHT

This pretty little wild herb is of great value for weakness of the sight, eye inflammation, colds affecting the eyes and hay fever. The infusion may be taken internally and used for bathing the eyes. Place an ounce of the herb in a pint of water which has boiled and cooled off a little. Allow to stand until cold. Dose: a small wineglassful three times daily. The homoeopaths prepare a fresh plant tincture from which an eye lotion can be made by mixing five drops in two tablespoonsful of rose water. Use this for sore and inflamed eyes; or employ the infusion. Homoeopathic Eyebright (Euphrasia) 3x may be used instead of the infusion for sore, inflamed eyes, colds and hay fever. Dose: five pills every three hours.

EYES

All homoeopathic chemists supply harmless and reliable eye drops for use in an eye bath or by means of an eye dropper. The nature of the drops depends on the condition to be treated, and the reader is urged to visit a homoeopathic practitioner and not experiment at home. Belladonna, Cineraria, Kali Iod. and Pulsatilla are examples of remedies used for this purpose. For harmless bathing purposes for sore, tired eyes, one cannot do better than to employ Eyebright (Euphrasia). (See also under **Honey**).

FAINTING

Keep the patient in the fresh air, loosen the clothing, sprinkle cold water over the face and hold a smelling bottle to the nose. If the patient is very prostrated give five drops of homoeopathic Moschus 3x every two hours. See also Collapse.

FASTING

All kinds of physical upsets (most of which have their origin in the stomach and bowels) can be cleared up without medicine. All the sufferer has to do is what an animal does by instinct when it is ill — go without food. Of course, this is far too simple to be tried by the majority of people, who have the erroneous idea firmly fixed in their minds that they will perish if they do not eat to 'keep up their strength'. Only a small portion of energy comes from food; the major supply is from the air. (See **Breathing** and **Diet**). When ill, the system is able to digest and assimilate hardly any food; or not any at all. So any food eaten is only a tax on the already depleted energy which is so urgently required to correct what is wrong in the system, and not to waste on getting rid of unwanted nourishment. Food eaten in such circumstances tends to turn foul and add to a toxic state already existing.

In some institutions prolonged fasts are undertaken for the treatment of even very serious ailments, and with marked success. But we must stress that prolonged fasts should be undertaken only under expert supervision. Even when taken under guidance a very long fast can, in some cases, do irreparable harm. Short fasts of two or three days, or even for a week, may be undertaken with decided benefit. On a fast the total resources of the organism are devoted to the most essential work in health restoration; namely, elimination of the toxic causes responsible for ill health. Poisons are rapidly elminated from the blood and tissues, and passed off through the usual channels.

Owing to this eliminative process the breath becomes foul, the tongue coated and bodily aroma unpleasant. There may be headaches, due to the liberated body poisons; and the faster may be low-spirited. As a rule, after the third day, all these unpleasant symptoms disappear. A 'hungry feeling' in the stomach passes. True hunger is eventually evidenced by a watering of the mouth, showing that the faster is ready to take food. If a week's fast is not considered, then even to go without food for one or two days will help the system, and is sufficient to throw off many acute conditions. To go without food for a single meal is all that is necessary to recitfy some stomach upsets.

During a fast take plenty of water. Drink it slowly. If

desired the water may be flavoured with fruit juices. Following a fast commence feeding on fruits and fresh salads. In some cases Slippery Elm food may be taken while abstaining from all other food except fruit juice. But as a rule it is better to avoid all nourishment unless taking Slippery Elm for curative purposes. Naturally, one has to use will power to go on a fast: that is what the will is for — to be made use of. Fasting helps to keep the body in subjection, hence the reason why it is a spiritual exercise. Anything demanding the use of the will builds character. It is wise when fasting to have an enema occasionally.

FATIGUE
See Anaemia, Collapse and Exhaustion. Also Bathing and Breathing.

FATS
Animal fats, and foods containing them, are bad for many people, especially those suffering from high blood pressure and arterial disorders. When the liver cannot deal properly with fats and oils that are of what is termed the 'saturated' type, the result leads to blood disorganisation, clots, arterial tension and heart trouble; also to ruptured capillaries and strokes. Margarine is prepared as a rule from natural, unsaturated oils; but these are 'processed' by a system which is the same as that which makes tallow candles, and the final product which reaches the table is harmful. Natural, unsaturated fats contain a larger percentage of iodine than the saturated variety.

Nut butters, from health food stores, are recommended. Use dairy butter sparingly. For cooking purposes sunflower seed oil, or maize oil, are very strongly recommended.

FEAR
There is an old saying that where the plague kills one, the fear of the plague kills ten. There is a great deal of truth in this. We are born in fear. The mother is often full of groundless fear and this mental state is transferred to the child. Indeed, psychologists agree that fear, or any kind of emotional upset, influences the unborn from the moment of conception. Fear continues to pester us from birth onwards,

and affects some far more than it does others. It clouds and darkens every phase of living. It may be said that all the negative emotions are nasty, withering forms of fear: hurry is fear of not having sufficient time; jealousy is fear of a rival; hate is usually due to inferior feelings and a fear that somebody else is better in some way, or has more of this world's goods; worry is fear that one cannot overcome difficulties, and so on. Fear is the worst enemy of mankind, and is behind wars and rumours of wars.

Diseases of mind and body can be caused by fear. If father died of cancer of the liver, and the daughter has a pain later on in life in the same region and with somewhat similar symptoms, she fears she has what father had. The thought takes root and she becomes sure of it. She is even afraid to go and have the condition diagnosed in case her fear is justified. In time the body cells take on the pattern of the fear thoughts, and a cancer is formed. Ninety-nine times out of a hundred this pain was originally nothing more than a congested liver, or some gall bladder trouble. Proper attention would have helped to remove the ungrounded fear and saved years of suffering.

This is not idle chatter; fear has caused cancer, even as it has caused a variety of physical disorders too numerous to mention. To eliminate fear, become a well-adjusted person, and enjoy living, read what we have to say on **Psychology** and **Spiritual aid.** To conquer fear is the first step to a new life.

> 'Tender-handed stroke a nettle,
> And it stings you for your pains:
> Grasp it like a man of mettle,
> And it soft as silk remains.'
>
> (Aaron Hill)

FEET

In ancient times a great deal of attention was given to the feet. Sore, painful and disfigured feet make standing or walking in the correct posture impossible. Wrong posture throws the spine out of position, and faults in the spine result in congested or impinged spinal nerves, which, in turn, means a sub-normal supply of nervous energy to body organs, and poor function. Or, the nerves may be irritated, resulting in organ upset.

High heels are responsible for many physical troubles in women, especially disorders of the reproductive organs: painful periods, irregularities, prolapse of the uterus, etc. Pinched feet set up great nervous irritation and cause mental tension, irritability, bad temper and morbidness.

Chinese healing and Zone Therapy prove that the condition of the feet greatly influences the body as a whole. Bodily disorders are registered in the feet by reflexes, and it is possible to diagnose a faulty organ by finding the corresponding sore or tender spot in the feet. By treating the sore spot with Massage, Acupuncture or hot Bathing the faulty organs are treated through the reflexes along the body zones.

The feet should be warm, and the head cool. When the reverse is present there exists circulatory imbalance and some sort of physical debility or illness. This is why a foot bath will help to cure colds, congestive headaches and various bodily upsets. Such baths aid in equalizing the circulation, drawing the congestion downwards from the brain and aiding the heart's action.

The feet should be washed daily. After drying it is good to massage the feet. Any kind of rubbing is helpful. Twist the feet, and stretch the toes — loosen them up. If you find any tender spots on the soles, the toe tops, or the sides of the feet, rub the areas vigorously with the finger tips.

For health's sake, change the hose frequently. Do not wear black hosiery.

Rheumatic suffers will be helped by adding a heaped teaspoonful of Epsom salts to a hot foot-bath. Acids will be eliminated through the large pores in the soles.

For sore, aching feet add a dessertspoonful of powdered boracic acid to the hot water; also sprinkle a little of the powder in the hose every morning. This is good for sweaty feet.

It is said that to give the soles of the feet a few rubs with a peeled clove of Garlic will aid in toxic elimination, help to cure coughs and colds and benefit the constitution generally.

Excessive foot-sweat points to toxaemia and/or debility. It is bad to suppress such sweating, as the body is getting rid of morbid matter in this manner. Remedies which often correct the cause of foot sweat without suppression are Sulphur and

Silica (homoeopathic). Sufferers may try Sulphur 30: five pills night and morning for two or three weeks. If results are not satisfactory try Silica 30 night and morning.

Much foot pain may be relieved by Arnica 3: four to five pills before meals three times daily. Distressing burning of the feet often responds to Apis Mel. 3: four or five pills before meals.

Cold feet point to circulatory troubles, or general debility. The remedy lies in finding and removing the cause, and building up a healthy organism. See also **Bathing, Breathing, Zone Therapy.**

FEMALE TROUBLES

Female irregularities are usually due to wrong living, self-abuse, worry and constitutional troubles. In many instances such troubles with married women are due to the abuse of sex; the husband usually being the responsible person. On the whole far too much stress is placed upon sex, resulting in a general depletion of the system of both women and men. Companionship between two people with similar ideals and view-points form the basis for ideal marriage; and happy companionships are frequently ruined by over-indulgence in sex. See also other headings: **Menstrual Disorders, Impotence, Menopause, Pregnancy, Uterus Prolapse** and **Marriage.**

When a woman has a pain in the breast, or she feels a lump there, it does not necessarily mean that she has a malignant condition. More often than not the 'lump' is nothing more than a matted, congested condition of the tissues. Massage the breasts with warm Olive oil night and morning, using a circular movement, and kneading the breasts gently. Paying attention to right living and wise thinking, and using common sense over sex matters will often result in such trouble clearing up.

Excellent homoeopathic remedies for breast troubles are Conium Mac. 30: four or five pills on rising, and Phytolacca 30: four or five pills on retiring. Scores of cases of breast trouble have cleared up by taking these two remedies for a few weeks. One celebrated homoeopathic physician says that, in his experience, they never fail. However, if breast pains persist it is sensible to visit a practitioner for diagnosis. To seek aid does not mean you are heading for an operation.

Sore nipples in nursing mothers are helped by applying a pinch of powdered Acacia before or after nursing (See **Acacia**).

FEVERS

Yarrow	½ ounce
Scullcap	½ ounce
Peruvian bark	½ ounce
Boneset	½ ounce

Simmer in two pints of water in an iron or enamel pot for fifteen minutes. The value will be increased if a teaspoonful of Composition Powder has been added; or, a little Cinnamon. Dose: a tablespoonful to a large wineglassful every two or three hours. May be flavoured with Lemon and Honey, or with Molasses or Liquorice. This herbal tea will control most fevers, eliminate the causes and add to bodily strength. It also calms the nerves. For the more serious fevers it is wise to seek professional aid. See also **Influenza** and the various headings, including **Bathing**.

A fever is an effort on the part of nature to 'burn up' accumlated waste matter. It may be controlled, but never suppressed.

Useful homoeopathic remedies for simple fevers are: Aconitum 3: Four pills every hour. If the sufferer does not improve within twelve hours the remedy should be discontinued. If there is a chill on the liver give five drops of Baptisia 1x every two hours. For the fevers of children Gelsemium 3 is a wonderful remedy: three or four pills every two hours. Another effective remedy, especially when the child is irritable, is Chamomilla 3: three or four pills every two hours. These remedies apply to the more simple types of fever, although both Baptisia and Gelsemium are helpful in Influenza.

The biochemic tissue salts, Ferr. Phos. and Kali Mur. 3x or 6x have done excellent work in feverish conditions of all types. Dissolve six or eight tablets of each in half a cup of hot water and give a teaspoonful every hour.

FIGS

Figs are excellent purifiers of the blood. One of the oldest cures recorded is that of King Hezekiah, who had a nasty boil. Speaking as the mouthpiece of Jehovah, Isaiah the prophet told the king to make a fig poultice and lay it on the boil. This was done, and the king recovered. So we have divine authority for the use of figs for boils and carbuncles. The fig cure is most effective, not only for boils, but for skin sores and septic conditions. The figs may be used as purchased, split and applied as a cold poultice; or, put some into an enamel pot and cover with new milk. Mash the figs slightly with a fork and apply as a poultice, as hot as the patient can bear. Also, drink about a cupful of the milk in which the figs have been simmered every day. The fig poultice should be large enough to cover the sore, and changed four times every twenty-four hours.

FIRST AID

See **Artificial Respiration, Haemorrhage, Wounds**. See also under **Collapse**.

FLATULENCE

Rapid eating and over-feeding will cause flatulence. To go without a meal will often be all that is necessary to correct the cause. A teaspoonful of Compound Tincture of Cardamoms in a little hot water is a grand medicine, and may be taken at any time. Reliable homoeopathic medicines are Nux Mosch. 3, Carbo Veg. 6, Asafoetida 3 and Valerian 3. Take five pills every fifteen minutes until the necessary relief has been obtained. This applies to whichever remedy is chosen. Or, take Nux. Mosch. before meals and Carbo Veg. after meals for a time to remove causes other than poor mastication. When the cause is nervous take Asafoetida before and Valerian after meals. All these remedies are of untold value to sufferers from indigestion and flatulence. See also **Indigestion, Diet**, etc.

FRACTURES

See remarks under **Comfrey**.

FRECKLES

Homoeopathic Sepia 30 or Primula Obconca 30 may be tried. If one fails try the other in about two weeks time. Take three or four pills of the selected remedy nightly.

A lotion of one part glycerine to two of lemon juice may be gently massaged into the areas once or twice daily. Equal parts of fresh milk and lemon juice may also be tried as a lotion.

FREEDOM

Human beings love freedom, but many get satisfaction by restricting the freedom of others. Authoritative institutions, political, religious and medical often greatly restrict the freedom of those outside their particular fences and of their own members.

Take, for example, the position in orthodox medicine. Within the ranks a doctor has to keep to a rigid code of ethics, and rightly so. Yet, in the opinion of many thinking people, some of the rules and regulations deter wise doctors from giving helpful information to the public and restrict them in the humane side of their work. We understand that a doctor is not permitted to associate professionally with any unorthodox healer however worthy he might consider his methods. He must keep within the fence.

Professional restrictions are so strong that if an unorthodox healer were to discover a cure for, say cancer, it would not be considered worthy of consideration. As one medical man said to the writer, 'Any cure for cancer or anything else must come from within the ranks of our (orthodox) medical profession, or from recognised (orthodox) scientists'. This means that the authoratitive institution of medicine holds itself up as a god. Good in matters medical must come from the one omnipotent source, and people could die by the thousand before doctors dare condescend to even consider a possible cure from elsewhere. It is regrettable that unorthodox organizations tend to follow in orthodox footsteps; they also build fences which members must keep within.

In religion the position is as bad. We learn of what the Bible calls 'the glorious liberty of the sons of God', but we fail to find it. If one dares to think for oneself and obey the divine invitation, 'Come, let us reason together', one is a crank and an enemy of truth. We are told that 'the truth shall make us free'. The old, old question is asked again and again: what is truth? Religionists should remember that Christ said 'I am the Way, the Truth and the Life'. He is Truth, and he said, 'By *this* shall all men know that ye are my disciples, in *that ye have love, one for another*'. St. Paul clearly points out that no matter what our knowledge may be, that even if we understand all mysteries and have all faith — even become a martyr, without love as the guiding principle it profits us nothing. So love is the divine measuring rod. Love brings freedom, and God *is* love. We are forced to conclude that those who profess to know the most about matters spiritual have failed to grasp the very fundamental teaching of the Master. Guns, bombs and battleships are blessed by priests in the name of the Prince of Peace. Shame! Those who try to be guided by the law of love are regarded as weak cranks, parasites and fools. But was not the founder of Christianity regarded in the same way?

As to political freedom — that's a case of 'Thus far shalt thou go, and no further'. Those who believe in the brotherhood of man and the common union of the people (That is what Communism literally means — common-union) seem to show even less brotherhood and freedom than those of other political colours.

Selfishness and greed manifest in all parties. Face the fact: most capitalists are greedy; and, once the socialist improves his lot he tends to want to hold on to what he has, get more and leans toward conservatism. True, there are intelligent and well-meaning men in all groups; but, for the majority, 'me and mine' is the rule. Humanity has a very poor idea of what universal brotherhood means, and what is not in the heart and mind cannot be expressed in living.

The truth is that there is a great deal of rubbish talked about freedom. It is almost impossible for any human organization to exist without regulations, and the imposition of laws and regulations is bound to limit freedom.

We hear of the freedom of the press. Unfortunately in many instances this means the freedom of editors and writers to distort facts, and to injure and sometimes destroy innocent souls. How often are innocent relatives of some person who has done wrong made to suffer mental agony in the columns of sensational newspapers! Fortunately newspapers also have the freedom to build, educate and help. It is obvious that freedom means the freedom to do the right, and not to indulge in wrong doing.

Everything in nature is governed by law, and real freedom is enjoyed when those fundamental laws are fully obeyed. The trouble in human society is that the laws themselves are often wrong, and not based on justice and human dignity.

Real freedom lies in being bound to principle. Any other kind of freedom is an illusion. Perfect freedom is that which springs from selfless Love — day to day living based on the standards set down by the One who was the Way and the Truth.

This subject of freedom has been mentioned because we find scores of people suffering from mental and physical maladies due entirely to frustrations set up by fear of authoritative institutions of one kind and another. To give one example: the writer has had many cases of neurosis caused by a fear that if the sufferer did not think exactly as he had been instructed to think by his religious organisation he was doomed. His reason caused him to have other views on certain matters; views which he dared not express. This state of mind is one that can and does produce quite serious illness. If what we are associated with causes fear, then something is wrong. God is Love; Love casts out fear; so any teaching based on fear is not of God. All must be free to worship in their own way according to the dictates of personal conscience. Fear nothing. God alone is the judge, and not any man-made organisation that has taken unto itself authority which belongs to God alone.

Live to principle to the best of your ability, and 'render unto Caesar the things that are Caesar's'; but be ready to suffer for the freedom to think and live according to your principles. When you have a free mind you will have a free body, and a free organism means a healthy, active mechanism. The body cannot be freed from disorders when the mind is tied up with fear. Be free!

GALL STONES

Three homoeopathic medicines are advised: Berberis

Vulgaris 30, Hura Braz. 30 and Cholesterin 30. Take five pills of Berberis 30 on rising, five of Cholesterin half an hour before lunch and five of Hura Braz. on retiring. We have witnessed spectacular results from this treatment after a few weeks. Some may prefer to take the potencies lower. If the third is favoured, take a dose of Berberis 3 and Cholesterin 3 before meals, and a dose of Hura Braz. 3 after meals, three times daily.

To ease the pain apply hot Fomentations over the area, and take some Olive oil. This brings us to what is known as 'the Olive oil cure'. Get half a pint of Olive oil and the juice of six Lemons. First, take a dose of Epsom salts. One hour later take a wineglassful of Olive oil followed immediately by a drink of Lemon juice; after five minutes repeat the procedure until all the oil has been taken. Take any remaining Lemon juice. The latter helps to retain the oil and prevent sickness. It is claimed that the stones soften and come away without pain. Others claim that all that comes away is congealed masses of oil. Practitioners say that X-ray photographs taken after the oil treatment show that it has been successful. The writer has reason to believe that the stones are removed by this method, but lacks conclusive proof. Anyway, this rather drastic treatment always brings great relief, and is well worth trying when other methods fail. Emulsified oil taken regularly is also said to prevent and cure gall stones (See Olive Oil).

A good herbal remedy is the fluid extract of Parsley Piert. One teaspoonful in a cup of hot water after meals three times daily for several weeks. On this treatment a dose of Epsom salts should be taken every morning. Leave the purgative alone as soon as results have been attained. The value of the homoeopathic treatment first mentioned is that purgatives are not called for.

GARLIC

Garlic cloves, cut up and covered with brown sugar or Honey, produce a syrup that is most beneficial for colds and coughs of all types. Give one or two teaspoonsful every hour. Garlic is an ancient remedy for auto-toxaemia and blood disorders, as well as for respiratory complaints. Highly diluted oil of Garlic is strongly advocated by nature cure enthusiasts and unorthodox healers. Its value is hard to over-estimate, as it certainly deals with toxic conditions of the intestines. Taken in capsule form there is no unpleasant aroma. Garlic does not cure everything, as some would have us believe. In a few cases it causes upset.

GASTRITIS

Treat as for **Indigestion**. See also **Acacia, Slippery Elm, Diet** and **Fasting**.

GELSEMIUM

This remedy is advised only in homoeopathic form. It acts on several organs of the body and is excellent for the nerves, muscular weakness, influenza, some feverish conditions, measles, kidney complaints, poor circulation and general debility. We recommend it for home use in cases of neuralgia and muscular pains, fevers — especially the fevers of children, colds, influenza and nervous exhaustion. Take four or five pills of Gelsemium 3 three times daily; for acute pain take a dose every hour. Gelsemium should also be taken hourly for influenza, although attention is drawn to the remarks given under **Influenza**. For the feverish colds of the very young Gelsemium is a grand remedy.

GEMS (CURATIVE)

To intelligent people, healing by means of precious stones may suggest superstition, witchcraft and hocus-pocus. Such will be surprised to learn that a very celebrated physician wrote a volume of nearly five hundred pages on *Precious Stones (Curative)* in 1907. We refer to Dr. W.T. Fernie. This book is now out of print. Dr. B. Bhattacharyya, a well known Indian scholar and a very learned man, has also written much on healing by the employment of gems. Some modern doctors have been broadminded enough to take up his teachings, and have investigated his work.

Healing with precious stones is a very ancient art. The Hebrew peoples, probably more than any other race, used gems for curative purposes. Gems were also used as symbols in religious rites. The breastplate worn by the high priest over his robes of glory and beauty consisted of twelve precious stones.

Says Dr. Fernie: 'Gems and precious stones retain within themselves a faithful and accurate record, even to the smallest detail, of physical conditions and acquired properties, from the primitive time of their original molecular beginning – the precious stone in us will continue to assert meantime its long-remembered virtues – for welfare (or the reverse) – '. Many gems have been processed in the chemistry of nature from the early days of earth's physical history; they have been formed, processed and subjected to enormous pressures, great heat and cosmic influences.

Colour plays a large part in health and disease, and today much interest is being shown in colour healing. It is known that colours from the red end of the spectrum vitalize, and sometimes irritate; the colours of the middle band are more neutral, but aid the middle of the body, normalizing the digestive and assimilative organs; colours from the blue end of the spectrum are sedative. It is most interesting to note that flowers with a yellow blossom tend to act on the liver and digestion, while blue flowers are sedative and nervine. Examples of the first (yellow) are Celandine, Dandelion and Berberis. These plants, bearing yellow blossoms, are all powerful activators of the stomach, liver and pancreas. Examples of plants bearing blue flowers are Scullcap, Baptisia and Vervain. These are excellent nerve remedies, and exert a very soothing influence on the brain and nervous system.

It is found that the colours of gems act in a similar manner: the ruby is stimulating; the emerald is neutral, and acts on the middle section of the organism; the sapphire is sedative and acts on the nervous system. Colours in plants and gems are due to the presence of minerals and it has been worked out that the minerals responsible for colours in the mineral and plant kingdoms also have a corresponding effect on the physical body, and even on the mind.

We must conclude that the ancient idea of certain gems warding off disease, when worn, has an element of truth in it.

Long, long ago, Eastern physicians gave finely powdered gems as medicine, and they do so till this day. Dr. Bhattacharyya has a method of making homoeopathic medicine from gems. Some medical men have investigated this method, and the results obtained prove beyond all doubt that great curative virtues reside in these decorative products of nature. The writer also endorses this discovery, having had some co-operation with Dr. Bhattacharyya and Dr. Beach of the U.S.A.

That the wearing of certain precious stones as ornaments can have helpful or harmful effects to the wearer, according to conditions, has also been confirmed. To quote Dr. Bhattacharyya: 'Mr. Joshi, a jeweller of Bombay, was advised by his friends to wear a ruby to increase his business (for the stimulating effect, we imagine?) — Mr. Joshi selected a powerful ruby of bright crimson colour, heavy in weight and full of lustre and brilliance. For the first three months nothing happened. But at the end of that period he developed a very high temperature. As usual, doctors were called in — strong pills were given to reduce the temperature, and immediately afterwards there was a collapse — when stimulants were administered, the patient regained consciousness, but discovered that his lower limbs were paralysed ...
Then started a series of treatments with stimulants, tonics, rays, electric charges and shocks, but nothing could help him. For nearly two years he remained paralysed — and was having a constant temperature. He became weak and emaciated.' The doctor goes on to describe other treatments which aided the paralysis, but did not touch the high temperature. Then Dr. Bhattacharyya saw the ruby, and the sufferer was asked to remove it from his person, and from the house. No medicine of any kind was given. The doctor continues: 'All were wonderstruck to find that his two-year-old temperature vanished within twenty-four hours. For ten years thereafter he had no temperature, and his health became so robust that it was difficult to recognise him ...'

This brief discussion on Gem Therapy has been included because of its interest. It goes to show that very powerful forces are locked up in the products of mother earth, and that old ideas should not be dismissed without a full investigation. See also Laws of Correspondence.

GENTIAN

The action and uses of this very old and deservedly popular simple tonic, appetizer and digestive are somewhat similar to Agrimony. The root is the part mostly employed medicinally. Simmer an ounce of the crushed root in a pint of water for half an hour. Strain. Dose: a small wineglassful before meals. May be flavoured with Liquorice; or, well sweetened with Honey to taste. Very fine for the digestion.

GINGER

Ginger root is carminative, stimulating and aids expectoration. Hence, it is good for indigestion, chills, debility and coughs. Given on its own it is quite effective, but it is usually mixed with other medicines. One quarter of a small teaspoonful in hot water, well sweetened, will usually relieve a disordered stomach and dispel flatulence. Added to any herbel tea for indigestion or colds, it will improve the action. In some respects it is similar to Cayenne, but is not so powerful a stimulant.

GINSENG

A Chinese remedy for debility, loss of appetite and nervous exhaustion. The dose is about fifteen grains of the powdered root immediately after meals. Wonderful medicinal virtues are supposed to exist in Ginseng, but we rather think that it does more for people who live where the plant grows than it does for those of other countries. In many respects this is true of a number of medicinal plants. Nature provides what is best suited to a sufferer in the area in which he resides.

GOITRE

Tincture of Oak bark	4 ounces
Tincture of Calendula	4 ounces
Tincture of Iodine	20 drops

This mixture may be taken internally, and used locally as a dressing. As a medicine take ten drops in an eggcup of cold water before meals, three times daily. More than this is not necessary.

A small folded handkerchief, soaked in the solution, may be applied to the goitre and kept on all night. Do not bind it in position tightly. Nothing tight must ever be applied to the throat.

Another method of treatment is to take five pills of homoeopathic Equisetum 30. on rising, and five of Iodine 30.

on retiring. Locally, gently massage Colloidal Iodine or 'Iodex' (from chemists) into the goitre at night.

GOLDEN ROD

In homoeopathic form, this is a fine remedy for hay fever. Take four or five pills of Solidago (the botanic name for Golden Rod) in the 12th potency morning and night. Some cases of hay fever require other remedies.

GOLDEN SEAL

The botanic name is Hydrastis. Five drops of the fluid extract in a little hot water before meals is a good remedy for indigestion, loss of appetite, nerviness and catarrh. However, quite a proportion of its virtue is lost in the making of the extract; the fresh plant tincture, as supplied by homoeopathic chemists, is far superior. It is expensive, but the dose for the fresh tincture need be only one drop in warm or cold water. Or, obtain it in the 30th. potency in pill form, and take four or five pills morning and night for a few weeks for any of the following troubles: catarrh, nervous debility, loss of appetite, indigestion, pain in the bowels, constipation, mucus accumulation in the throat, piles (some cases), soreness of the vagina, sore gums and mouth ulcers. Also good for catarrh of the Eustachian tubes. Hydrastis is one of those constitutional remedies which cover a very wide range, and can only do good. The root of the Gold Thread is somewhat similar, and this may be used when Hydrastis is not obtainable.

GOUT

Treat as for **Arthritis** or **Rheumatism**. Also give a kidney remedy such as Broom or Buchu. Homoeopathic Colchicum 30, one dose nightly, is an excellent remedy.

GRINDELIA

A very helpful remedy in the treatment of asthma. Also for coughs. May be taken in herbal or homoeopathic form. Five to ten drops of the fluid extract (according to age) in a little hot water, three times daily, is the usual dose. Or it may be added to other suitable remedies. Homoeopathically, we advise the 30th. potency: four or five pills on rising, and again on retiring.

GUAIACUM

Ten drops of the fluid extract of Guaiacum in hot water three times daily, cleanses the blood and is a very fine remedy for rheumatism and weakness of the capillaries. It has some value in cases of high blood pressure, helping to keep the small arteries healthy. It is also useful for sore mouth and tongue. It has gained quite a reputation in the treatment of obstinate blood and skin disorders.

May be taken homoeopathically for any of these ailments. Take four or five pills of the 3rd. potency before meals three times daily; or five of the 30th. potency morning and night.

GUMS

Sore, inflamed or spongy gums are helped by a mouth wash of one teaspoonful of Calendula (tincture) in a wineglass of cold water. Well wash the mouth with this three times daily. Guaiacum or Golden Seal are also helpful gum remedies. (See **Pyorrhoea**).

HAEMORRHAGE

Add a teaspoonful of distilled extract of Witch Hazel to half a tumbler of cold water and administer a teaspoonful every five minutes. Except for cases of simple Nose-bleed professional aid should be called immediately. Give the Witch Hazel until help arrives. Ferr. Phos., 3x or 6x, may be given additionally: three tablets every few minutes.

It is claimed by some authorities that haemophilia (bleeder's disease) is helped by eating peanuts regularly.

HAIR

Treat the scalp as stated under **Dandruff**, and remember that dead hair has to come away. Vigorous massage of the scalp simply causes dead hair to come out more quickly, so that new growth is aided.

Brush the hair frequently. Hair, like everything else to do with the body, depends on the quality of the blood for its health and lustre: so those with thin and falling hair must pay attention to sane living and dieting. We have often had patients with falling hair, partial baldness, scurf and early greying. These people have never come for hair treatment, but for other physical troubles. It has, however, been very noticeable, that as the physical disorders have been eliminated, and the general health improved, the hair has also responded. There has been new growth and new life in what the ladies regard as their 'crowning glory'.

Be careful of hair and scalp lotions. They can be very harmful to some people. Any hair lotion containing Bay Rum and Jaborandi should be valuable. Jaborandi is a real tonic to the hair roots. Any chemist can make up a lotion for the hair with these two items, and such a preparation cannot be bettered for general use as a hair dressing. But, when the scalp is much troubled with Dandruff the methods stated under that heading should be employed.

Gentle massage of the scalp with Castor oil at night, followed by a shampoo the next morning is recommended by some specialists. This should be done once or twice weekly.

Hair cannot grow, or be healthy, without Silica. So the sufferer from hair and scalp trouble is advised to take Silica 6x or 8x (from homoeopathic chemists). Dissolve two tablets on the tongue before meals three times daily for some weeks. A compound tablet composed of homoeopathic Calcium, Silica, Lycopodium, Jaborandi and Ceanothus is sold by some homoeopathic chemists. It is known as formula P.57. This compound remedy is helpful for all hair and scalp troubles, including anaemia of the scalp. It is also a good constitutional tonic. The dose is two tablets before meals three times daily.

HATE

Hate means fear, and these two in combination form the most destructive force in human society. "Love casts out fear'. 'Fear hath torment'. No sick person can get really well under treatment if he or she is troubled by hatred. Quite often the removal of hatred will result in the cure of a bodily disorder without any other treatment. Read what we have to say on Love, Psychology and Spiritual Aid.

HAWTHORN

The ripe fruit of the Hawthorn (Crataegus Oxycantha) is used in herbal and homoeopathic medicine as a heart remedy. It was introduced by a Dr. Green of Ireland, who had employed it with marked success in cases of heart failure and various disorders of that organ. Dr. John H. Clarke says that it is the nearest approach to a positive heart tonic. It is one of the few remedies that homoeopaths use in material doses as well as in potency, and we obtain excellent results from both.

The Hawthorn fruit is a positively harmless medicine. It not only strengthens the muscle and valves of the heart, but is of benefit in cases of dropsy, debility from sexual excesses, nervous debility and the irritability of disposition so often found in heart cases.

The dose is about ten drops of the fluid extract in a little hot water three times daily; but far better results will be obtained from the fresh plant tincture, as supplied by homoeopathic chemists. The dose for the fresh plant tincture is five to ten drops in hot or cold water, three times daily. Those who prefer to use it in potency may take five pills of the 3rd potency three times daily.

HAY FEVER

In our opinion, homoeopathic remedies are the best. The selection of the right remedy depends largely on what type of dust or pollen causes the upset. Probably the best general remedy is Sabadilla 30. Five pills morning and night; or, three times daily during a bout of the trouble. Other remedies are: Sambul, Moschus, Solidago, Sticta, Euphrasia, Anthoxantum, Allium Cepa. Any of these may be tried, and taken in the same manner as advised for Sabadilla. The remedies are given in what we consider to be their order of importance, but this does not necessarily apply in all cases, as sufferers differ so much. If one remedy fails, try another.

One may also try using powdered Bayberry bark as a snuff. The effect is to harden the membranes of the nose and render them less sensitive to irritating substances. It has proved most successful in some cases; but the user must be prepared for an attack of sneezing when using a snuff for the first few times. As one sufferer wrote: 'After a sniff I seemed to have several attacks of hay fever all at once. The next time it was not so bad. After a week I lost my symptoms, and have not had an attack since.' (See also under Honey).

HEADACHE

One may take away the pain with a suppressive drug; but that does not remove the cause. The choice of remedy depends on the type of headache. It may be congestive and partly due to blood pressure; it may be 'nervous', due to indigestion or to some organic trouble.

Congestive headaches are often removed by taking homoeopathic Glonoine 30. Four or five pills every fifteen minutes for three doeses, and then a dose morning and night for a period. Aconitum 30. (taken as for Glonoine) will cure some neuralgia type of headache, and so will Gelsemium or Chamomilla. The latter is also good for headaches due to digestive or nervous upset. A good general remedy that may be tried in all cases is Melilotus. Obtain the fresh plant tincture from a homoeopathic chemist. Take five drops in a little warm water every fifteen minutes until relief is obtained. Melilotus may also be inhaled.

A really hot Foot Bath, with the water well up over the ankles, will afford speedy relief in most cases of headache, no matter what the cause. Menthol ointment massaged into the temples, forehead and back of the neck is helpful. Also, insert a little into the nostrils. Hot towels to the anus has a magical effect with some (See **Bathing**).

Migraine headaches usually respond well to either homoeopathic Iris Ver.30. or to Onosmodium 30. When one fails try the other. The dose is five pills every half an hour, and then five morning and night for a time to remove the constitutional causes. Migraine cases need to build up their nervous and digestive systems. Spirits of Camphor, applied on a folded handkerchief to the back of the head and neck, give marked relief. This is also good for neuralgia of the face and neck.

HEART TROUBLE

There are several forms of heart disorder, and the condition should be diagnosed. All sufferers must feed sensibly to avoid indigestion. Many a cause of heart failure has been due to a badly upset stomach, and nothing else. Digitalis in material form, as given by the orthodox profession, has done good; but it has also harmed thousands of heart sufferers, and its frequent employment can damage the heart. Harmless remedies which replace Digitalis are **Lily of the Valley, Cactus Grandiflorus** and **Hawthorn** (See headings). All these are harmless.

The remedies may be taken in the form of fluid extracts, or as fresh plant tinctures, the latter being vastly superior. Here is a good formula which suits many heart cases, and which can do harm to none. It tones the heart muscle, strengthens the valvular action and improves the circulation:

Fluid extract Lily of the Valley	1 ounce
Fluid extract Cactus Grandiflorus	1 ounce
Fluid extract Hawthorn	1 ounce
Tincture of Cayenne	1 drachm

Dose: Ten to twenty drops in a little hot water before meals three times daily.

Fresh plant tinctures will be more expensive, but the dose need be only five to ten drops in warm or cold water, three times daily. If the reader wishes to get the formula in fresh plant tinctures from a homoeopathic chemist, ask for this:

Convallaria	½ ounce
Cactus Grand	½ ounce
Crataegus	½ ounce
Capsicum	30 mins.

Kali Phos.12. is also a fine heart tonic, and may be taken in addition to the above. Five pills on retiring nightly. There are many other heart remedies. The sufferer should avoid worry, and go to an experienced homoeopathic physician if he does not respond to home treatment. Worry plays havoc with the heart; indeed, all mental and emotional upsets interfere with the physical organ. There is even what we term 'psychological heart'. The experienced homoeopath can deal with all forms of heart trouble. Camphor is a heart stimulant. See also Angina.

HELLEBORE

Used homoeopathically, the Black Hellebore (Helleborous Nig.) is a reliable remedy for debility and melancholia, especially in females. Four or five pills of the 30th. potency morning and night for a while. Also good for amenorrhoea.

HELONIAS

Used homoeopathically this is a remedy of great power for prolapse of the uterus, ovarian pain, disorders of the mammary glands, fear and melancholia. Dose: Helonias 30. Four or five pills on rising and on retiring.

HEMLOCK

This is the poison taken by Socrates, and it should only be taken in homoeopathic potency, when it is quite harmless and a very wonderful medicine. It is prescribed for a number of ailments, but we suggest its use here for disorders of the female breast. When there is 'lumpiness', soreness and inflammation, take four or five pills of Hemlock 30. (Conium Mac.) on rising and on retiring. It is much better when taken alternately with Phytolacca 30. Take Conium Mac. 30. on rising, and Phytolacca 30. on retiring.

HENBANE

This is the Hyoscyamus of the homoeopaths. It is a great remedy for hysteria, especially in females. May be used by both sexes. For excitability, hysteria and great irritability take four or five pills of the 30th. potency morning and night. Helpful in many cases of rheumatism and arthritis.

HERBALISM

The most ancient of all systems of healing, and still one of the best. The modern skilled herbalist can produce cures when orthodox medicine has to resort to surgery. One must not associate the modern, highly trained botanic practitioner with the little shop in a back street of former days. There have always been great herbal physicians but never have they been better informed or as capable as they are today. The writer is acquainted with the type of training given by The National Institute of Medical Herbalists, and can say that those who receive a training from the Institute are capable diagnosticians and healers. King Henry the VIII granted the herbalists a charter. It is still in force! The above institute also boasts a Coat of Arms granted by the College of Arms.

Non-poisonous herbs work in harmony with the vital force of the organism. They are foods as well as medicine. They do not suppress, but elminate toxins, vitalize, restore and build in harmony with nature's laws.

Several herbs have been recommended for similar disorders, so that when one is not obtainable you can select what is available.

'The fruit of the tree shall be for food, and the leaf thereof for medicine'. (The Bible).

HERNIA (RUPTURE)

Gentle exercise under expert guidance can be most helpful in certain cases. Usually, a properly fitted truss is essential. To bring strength to the affected parts try taking one drop of distilled extract of Witch Hazel in a wineglassful of cold water before every meal. Another good remedy is homoeopathic Millifolium 3. Five pills after every meal. It will be necessary to keep up treatment for some time. A compress of Witch Hazel may be kept over the hernia every night. Much good has resulted from such compresses.

HERPES

The internal treatment should be as given under **Shingles**. Additionally for herpes of the lips dab with moist table salt two or three times daily.

HICCOUGH

This can be very distressing when it persists. Homoeopathic Mag.Phos.3x, six tablets in a wineglass of hot water, taken in sips, has proved successful. Here is an old country remedy that rarely fails: take a full drink of cold water and hold it in the mouth. Press the middle fingers in both ears and swallow the water, removing the fingers after a moment or two. Repeat if necessary. Why this acts we do not know. The fact remains that in most instances it is successful, no matter how the wise (?) laugh at the method.

Another strange cure is to exhale into a paper bag, and then to inhale from the bag one's own exhaled breath. It should be done quickly. In one country village they swallow a mouthful of mint sauce for hiccough, and claim it will cure.

A foot bath, foot manipulation or hot towels to the anus will sometimes be effective.

HOMOEOPATHY

John H. Clarke, M.D., a celebrated physician, and one of the most prolific writers on the science of medication, says of homoeopathy: '(It is) the most complete and scientific system of healing the world has ever seen'.

Homoeopathy is based on the law of similars. That is to

say 'like cures like'. Any medicine or drug taken in large material doses by a healthy person will produce certain disease symptoms; so any sufferer manifesting *similar symptoms* will be cured by taking an infinitesimal dose of that particular medicine which, in large doses, produces symptoms similar to the disease. For example: Belladonna is a poison in material doses. It produces fever, a flushed face, headache, etc. A sufferer with a fever and associated symptoms exactly similar to those caused by a healthy person taking crude Belladonna, can be cured by taking very minute doses of homoeopathically potentised Belladonna. It is common for drunkards to take a *little* alcohol in the morning after a bad night, to put them right. When a finger is burned accidentally, the burn will be healed more quickly and the smarting instantly relieved, if the finger is held for a very brief moment to a source of heat. Many illustrations of the homoeopathic law could be cited. Large doses of Quinine will cause fever of the malarial type. Minute doses will cure that type of fever; but only if the dose is very small.

Cutting up Onions causes the eyes to water and the nose to run. A cold, characterized by similar symptoms of watering of the eyes and nose, will be cured by potentised Onion. Sometimes even to smell an Onion will cure such colds, if it is done in time. But, be it noted, a cold with other symptoms will not respond to the Onion.

Dr. Hahnemann (the founder of homoeopathy) and many of his followers were helped in their researches by 'provers'. Provers were healthy people who offered their services for the testing of medicines and drugs. Some risked their lives by taking lethal doses of poisons, so that the effects could be carefully noted. For many years this 'proving of medicines' was undertaken, and the results carefully compiled into homoeopathic works on materia medica and repertories. 'Proving' is still done, although not to the same extent as there is now a vast number of 'proved' remedies. Two diseases of exactly the same nature cannot exist in the body at the same time, and the remedy which, in crude form, produces similar disease symptoms to those a patient manifests, cures the disease when it has been potentised. Hence, homoeopathy is based on natural laws.

Potentising is done by thoroughly shaking up one drop of

a crude medicine with ninety-nine drops of pure spirit. This is the first potency. Then one drop of the first potency is added to ninety-nine drops of spirit and the shaking process repeated. This goes on for three, six, thirty or even hundreds of times. The remarkable thing is that the more the remedy is split up the greater is its power. After the sixth potency it ceases to exist as a material substance, but becomes a powerful 'force' — the 'essence' or 'spirit' of the medicine. With minerals a method called trituration is involved for the first few processes, as shaking in spirit does not split up the molecules of a hard substance, and unless a medicinal substance is thoroughly split up it is of far less value and, in some instances, useless. One part of the mineral is mixed with nine parts of sugar of milk and pounded thoroughly for about two hours. This is the first trituration and is called 1x. One part of the 1x is then mixed with nine parts of milk sugar and the pounding (triturating) resumed. The process continues to the 6x trituration; after then, in most instances, spirit can be used and the potentising continued by the shaking method.

In homoeopathy (as in Schuessler Biochemistry) an 'x' following a figure denotes the degree of trituration (or potentisation) reached. Hence, a mineral or hard substance may be anything from 1x to 6x or even higher. Sometimes trituration is continued up to the 12x.

After the 6x is reached it is usual to continue the process by the liquid method as the substance is soluble.

A remedy name followed by a figure without an 'x' indicates that it has been prepared on the centesimal scale (one in 99 drops) although, on some occasions, a 'c' is shown after the figure.

Remedies with an 'x' following the number shows that the preparation has been carried out on the decimal scale (1 in 9). Some vegetable substances such as Lycopodium must be triturated up to 6x or more in order to break up the substance and liberate the full remedial force; shaking of the tincture alone in the first stages would result in a very imperfect medicine.

Pure homoeopathy is the employment of a single medicine which meets all the symptoms — the medicine which, by proving, has presented a perfect picture of the sufferer's ailments. This is the ideal method of Hahnemann. Many homoeopaths give more than one medicine, and some even give homoeopathic medicines in combination. One cannot deny the results obtained by the latter methods, although alternate medicines or mixtures are not homoeopathy in the real sense of the term. In all instances, unless liquids are prescribed, the little pills are dissolved on the tongue.

In skilled hands homoeopathy produces miracles of healing. Serum therapy and vaccinations are crude and harmful applications of the homoeopathic 'idea,' but out of harmony with the homoeopathic 'law.'

HONEY

'My son, eat thou honey, for it is good' (Solomon). Honey is a pure food and energiser. One of the best things a person can do for health's sake is to use Honey instead of sugar. Commercial sugar and sweets are most harmful; they do untold damage to the nerves, digestive and circulatory systems. On the other hand, Honey strengthens the heart, activates the endocrine glands and improves organic functions generally. A cup of hot water with a teaspoonful of Honey in it, gives immediate energy, and is superior to the much-advertised glucose. May be flavoured with Lemon if desired. A good pinch of red pepper increases its value as a natural stimulant.

Honey is helpful to all bronchial and hay-fever sufferers.

Those who do not care for Honey taken raw may try boiling a teaspoonful or so in water or milk. Taken thus it seems to suit some people better than raw Honey and for such is rather more curative.

Honey contains measurable traces of iron, copper and manganese, which are partly responsible for its remedial virtue. It is digested immediately it enters the stomach, so is no tax on the organism. Its constant use aids the kidneys and bowels; it is healing for inflamed states of the stomach and intestines, and the mucous surfaces everywhere. In hot milk or water it is ideal for sore throats, coughs and bronchitis. Locally it makes a fine ointment for sores, wounds and ulcers. It allays irritation and is good to apply to chapped hands. Will afford relief for frost-bite and will help to reduce swellings. A drop or two of liquid honey poured into inflamed eyes will usually give immediate relief. Honey mixed with fresh cream is said to be good for freckles. Spread on cloth it is a fine application for sore patches on skin, and also for Erysipelas. Many have found relief from piles by applying it regularly to the anus. But, the Honey must be pure, and not blended with glucose or sugar, if it is to be effective.

Some of the old herbalists regarded Honey as an elixir of life and a means for living to a good old age.

A teaspoonful boiled in half a pint of water for five minutes is grand for bathing sore and weak eyes. Bathe the eyes with the cold preparation two or three times daily. A Honey-water pack worn over the closed eyes at night is also of considerable benefit.

Apply Honey as an ointment for an inflamed or ulcerated cervix of the uterus. For this purpose it has proved to be effective when other means have failed. Apply with the finger, or on a wad of cotton wool pushed into position night and morning.

HOPS

A fine old remedy for nervousness and insomnia. Place an ounce of Hops in a pint of boiling water; keep covered and allow to cool off for half an hour. Dose: a wineglassful before or after meals, and again on retiring. Take warm for best effects. An old country custom was to stuff a pillow with Hops and sleep with the head resting on the pillow. Evidence is to hand showing that this helped to cure some bad cases of sleeplessness. Hop pillows may, in some instances, cause drowsiness during the day, especially when the individual is sensitive to the remedy.

HOREHOUND

Simmer an ounce in a pint of water, using an iron or enamel pan, for ten minutes. Strain. This is an excellent medicine for coughs and bronchitis. It also has some tonic value, and is not unpleasant to take. The dose is from a dessertspoonful to a tablespoonful for children, according to age, and rather more for adults. Take warm, three times daily.

HORSE CHESTNUT

Probably the best of all remedies for piles. May be used in fluid extract form, or homoeopathically. The dose for the fluid extract is five to ten drops in hot water before or after meals, three times daily. We favour the homoeopathic dilution. Ask for Aesculus Hip.30. Dose: five pills on rising and again on retiring. If necessary may be taken for several weeks.

HORSERADISH

The scraped fresh root is a good medicine for a weak stomach and kidneys. Has been found useful in dropsy. Take it sprinkled over salads or cooked meals. A medicine for indigestion and kidney trouble is prepared by pouring a pint of boiling water over an ounce of shredded root and half an ounce of crushed Mustard seed. After standing for an hour it is ready to take. Dose: a tablespoonful before every meal.

HORSETAIL

For years this grass has been considered an excellent remedy for dropsy and kidney troubles, incontinence of urine, gravel, irritation, etc. It is also given for acidity. The late Dr. Guyon Richards discovered that when given homoeopathically, it was one of the best remedies for an over-active thyroid, and had excellent effects on excitable and 'nervy' people. The dose is five pills morning and night. Ask for Equisetum 30. The infusion, or fluid extract, is good for kidney ailments, but does not appear to have any marked effect on the thyroid. The infusion is one ounce of the herb to a pint of water taken in small wineglassful doses three times daily; or half a small teaspoonful of the fluid extract in warm water.

HOUSEMAID'S KNEE

Complete rest is necessary. Locally, apply a compress of distilled extract of Witch Hazel, and renew three or four times daily. A compress may be kept on all night. Internally, take two tablets of Silica 6x or 8x before meals, and five pills of Rhus Tox. 3. after meals.

HYDROCOTYLE

This is one of the Asiatic remedies for which great claims are made, and it probably does more for people living in the East than it does for those living in the Western world. It is helpful in fevers, blood disorders, kidney weakness and skin complaints, especially the latter. We recommend it in the 30th. potency (homoeopathic) for skin diseases. Four or five pills morning and night. May be tried when other remedies fail.

HYSSOP

Like Horehound, this is an excellent medicine for respiratory troubles of every type. It is usually blended with other herbs, although it is quite effective on its own. It is best taken as an infusion. Simmer an ounce in a pint of water for twenty minutes. Strain. Flavour with Liquorice or Honey if desired. Dose: a dessertspoonful to a wineglassful, according to age, three or four times daily.

HYSTERIA

Homoeopathic Hyoscyamus 30. is probably the best remedy. Other good remedies are Ignatia 30., Natrum Mur. 30., Aurum Nat. Mur. 30. and Asafoetida 30. Read up these remedies in a homoeopathic repertory and make the selection according to individual symptoms. In most cases Hyoscyamus will act. During an attack give five pills every ten minutes. Otherwise, a dose morning and night for a short period to help remove causes. Herbal teas which are valuable in these cases are Scullcap, Valerian and Chamomile. The ordinary tincture of Asafoetida is also most helpful, the dose being three drops in water three times daily before meals. If the cause is an over-active thyroid, give Equisetum 30. Hot Foot Baths, or Hot Towels to the anus are always helpful. Also, bathing the head in cold water.

IGNATIA

St. Ignatius beans should be used homoeopathically. In many respects this remedy is similar in its effect to Nux Vomica, but it works in a different manner. Nux Vomica seems to act mainly on the physical, while Ignatia works through the psyche. Some writers say that Nux Vomica is a male medicine, and that Ignatia is a female remedy. Experience shows that, when correctly prescribed, it is a powerful medicine for both sexes. It acts on the mind, being good for hysteria or silent grief, troubles resulting from love affairs and nervous upsets. It has produced excellent results in affections of the throat and kidneys. The sufferer requiring Ignatia is always changing, both mentally and physicaly. It is a remedy to be considered in hyper-sensitive cases. May be given in the 6th. or 30th. potency, although better results follow the 30th. as a rule.

Give four or five pills of Ignatia 30. morning and night for moodiness, hysteria, grief, throat affections, kidney weakness, constipation, prolapse of the uterus or rectal muscle and coughs which are aggravated by coughing. Noise, touch and other people always aggravate an Ignatia patient. Be guided by the mental symptoms. Sufferers are worse in the morning, for taking coffee and smoking. Meals tend to upset, although they are better while actually eating.

Ignatia can be most helpful in cases of disorganized blood and arterial diseases.

IMPOTENCE

Impotence may be due to general debility, endocrine gladular imbalance, hormone deficiency, or to psychological causes. It is a great mistake to try to stimulate the sexual function by taking any kind of stimulant. Many of these sex-stimulators are sold in the chemists, and they are often dangerous. When the sex function is weak, or has 'packed up', it is obvious that nature needs a rest. To take stimulants in such circumstances will be at the expense of the general vitality, and the sufferer will become weaker in the end. Sexual debility is, naturally, a worry to both sexes; especially to men. The way to invite impotency is to fear it, and worry over sex will soon reduce a sexually weak individual to total impotency. The first essential in such cases is to try and forget sex for a time, and give the body a chance to build up. This alone will bring about a cure in some cases. What usually happens is that the sufferer keeps on indulging in sex, and often in self-abuse, to try and convince himself that his power is returning, thus weakening himself still further.

To-day many doctors are so obsessed with the teaching of Freud that in their anxiety to prescribe freedom for the individual, and in view of the obvious harm caused by frustration, proclaim that no harm is caused by masturbation if the individual is guilt-free.

This contention is not based on fact and observation. On the whole homoeopathic doctors, who study individuals more than diseases, disagree with this nonsense concerning total freedom over sexual matters. The results of prolonged masturbation are so very obvious, irrespective of the mental factor. A long life of experience has proved to the writer that the practice of uncontrolled masturbation causes harm to both mind and body. It is merely a matter of common sense. See remarks under **Marriage**.

Many diseases can be traced to sexual indulgence, but a feeling of guilt over sexual matters may be even worse than the indulgence. The sufferer should read what we have to say on **Psychology** and **Spiritual Aid**. Exercise, deep breathing and sane living will do much to restore normal function. Get interested in things outside the self. Indulge in games, club activities or some creative hobby. When the mind becomes obsessed with sexual thoughts, splash the organs with cold water, which will take away the desire and also tone the organs. It cannot be stressed too much that self-help in these cases is of paramount importance.

Here are some helpful remedies: take five pills of Staphisagria 30. on rising, and five of Nat. Mur. 30. on retiring, for a few weeks. Also a dose of Ignatia 30. occasionally, if the mind is much upset. If no results from Staphisagria and Nat. Mur., try Hydrocotyle 30. on rising, and Dirca 30. on retiring.

When there has been sexual frustration take Nux Vom. 30. morning and night for a week or two. A fear that a *lack* of sex has caused harm will be helped by Lachesis 30. morning and night. Sexual frigidity has been helped by taking Hydrocotyle 30. twice daily, while a feeling of sexual inferiority may be dispelled by taking Platina 30. on rising and Silica 30. on retiring. Other good remedies for sexual debility are Agnus Castus, Actaea Race., and Caladium. Agnus and Caladium are especially good in cases of masturbation. Staphisagria is, perhaps, the best general remedy, and may be tried first. The reader will be helped by consulting a homoeopathic repertory. Remember, remedies can do little unless the mind controls the body; but, with co-operation, remedies can produce most satisfactory results.

When the above remedies fail try homoeopathic Damiana Φ. Five drops in a little cold water before breakfast and dinner for a few weeks.

Another fine medicine is the fluid extract of Black Willow (Salix Nigra). Fifteen to twenty drops in a little hot water before meals, three times daily.

INCONTINENCE OF URINE

Homoeopathic Belladonna 3. Four pills before meals. If that fails try Apis Mel. 3. Two tablets of Ferr. Phos. 6x after meals may also help. There are several remedies, and any which improves the tone of the kidneys and bladder should be helpful. See the information given under those headings. Frequent urination due to prostate troubles call for Prostate Gland remedies.

INDIGESTION

A doctor with a reputation for curing indigestion said that this disorder was at the back of all ailments. Of course he was very wrong, but there is a measure of truth in the statement. The food makes the blood, and the blood is the life; so if the mechanism which deals with the food is out of order, it follows that the blood and all bodily organs must suffer as a result. However, there are other causes behind indigestion and the condition of the stomach may be a result of a morbid state of mind and wrong living in general. In other words, it is not so much the indigestion, but what causes it.

Sufferers should pay attention to diet, bathing, breathing, etc. The information given under Diet is vitally important. The most important rules are to eat only when hungry, partake of plain, natural foods and to well masticate everything.

There are dozens of excellent remedies, both herbal and homoeopathic. Here is a fine herbal recipe:

Agrimony	½ ounce
Crushed Dandelion root	½ ounce
Chamomile flowers	½ ounce
Centaury	½ ounce

Simmer gently in two pints of water in an iron or enamel pot for fifteen minutes, keeping the lid on. Strain, and add four ounces of Compound Tincture of Cardamoms and a tablespoonful or more of Honey. Stir thoroughly. Dose: one tablespoonful before every meal. Children less according to age. The substitution of Gentian root and Peruvian bark for Dandelion and Centaury (same quantities) will suit some cases better, especially if there is marked general debility. If Gentian and Peruvian bark are used, simmer for twenty minutes.

Homoeopathic Nux Vomica 3. is a wonderful remedy for indigestion, especially for tired, over-worked business men. All cases can try Nux Vom. of course. Ignatia 6. may suit ladies better than Nux Vom. Bismuth 6. will meet the requirements of others. Dosage of each remedy five pills before meals three times daily. The taking of crude Bismuth and soda preparations over long periods will tend to ruin any stomach. If the liver is much at fault, see **Liver** disorders. If troubled with flatulence, see under **Flatulence**. An emetic will almost certainly end a bout of acute indigestion.

INFANTS TROUBLES

Homoeopathic Chamomilla 3. is a grand remedy for peevish, irritable infants. Excellent for tummy troubles, wind and pain associated with teething. Obtain the remedy in liquid form, and give two or three drops in a feed twice daily; or administer in a teaspoonful of milk.

Calc. Phos. 3x is also fine for teething children. May be given in addition to Chamomilla: two tablets crushed and added to feeds two or three times daily; or given in a teaspoonful of milk or water.

Chamomilla will soothe the nervous system and quieten the mind. Calc. Phos. will give strength to bones and teeth.

When baby is very acid give two tablets of Nat. Phos. 3x in feeds two or three times daily. See also **Teething**.

INFLUENZA

Elder flowers	½ ounce
Boneset	½ ounce
Peppermint	½ ounce

| Cinnamon (rubbed) | ½ ounce |
| Composition powder | 1 teaspoonful |

Simmer in two pints of water, in an iron or enamel pot, for fifteen minutes, keeping the lid on. Strain. Keep the patient in bed and give a wineglassful, hot, every two hours. Children less according to age. May be sweetened with pure Honey. Avoid food until the temperature has dropped. As a beverage give plenty of diluted fresh Lemon juice with Honey, to which a pinch of Cinnamon may be added.

Homoeopathic remedies include Baptisia 30., Gelsemium 30. and Cinnamon 30. If not taking the herbal tea, give five pills of Cinnamon 30. every two hours, and either Baptisia 30. or Gelsemium 30. between the does of Cinnamon – thus: Cinnamon at 8 a.m., Gelsemium at 9 a.m., Cinnamon at 10 a.m., Gelsemium at 11 a.m., and so on. As the patient improves reduce the frequency of the doses.

The finest homoeopathic remedy of which we know is Cadmium Sulph. This remedy was used for certain types of fever and exhaustion for many years. Dr. Guyon Richards discovered its undoubted value in Influenza. Taken alternately with Cinnamon it kills the 'flu virus (A or B type). Cadmium Sulph. also removes the great depression associated with this fever. We have never known it to fail. The astonishing fact is, that after taking Cadmium Sulph. for Influenza, people who have suffered from severe bouts of this trouble year after year, often cease to be troubled again. In just a few cases there has been a return, but we have not heard of a return for a second time. The banishment of the tendency to Influenza appears to take place only when the remedy is given in very high potency. Lower potencies help greatly to promote a cure, but they act more slowly than the high potencies, and do not seem to prevent further attacks when 'flu is about.

The C.M. potency of Cadmium Sulph. is recommended, and the 200th. potency of Cinnamon. Take five pills of Cadmium Sulph. C.M. at 8 a.m., and five of Cinnamon 200. at 10 a.m. Then five of Cadmium Sulph. at 12 noon, and five of Cinnamon at 2 p.m. Continue the remedies, alternately, every two hours throughout the day, and also the day following if the symptoms are still present. After the second

THE NATURAL HOME PHYSICIAN 141

day, if some symptoms remain, drop the potency of Cadmium Sulph. to the 30th., and the same with the Cinnamon. As a rule further treatment will not be necessary. During the treatment plenty of hot Lemon and Honey may be taken.

The herbal or either of the homoeopathic methods will prove successful, as we have witnessed time and time again; but there is no doubt that the use of the high potency Cadmium Sulph. and Cinnamon is one of the greatest discoveries in medicine. Treatment is harmless. It is a great shame that the orthodox medical profession laughs at the idea of such high potencies curing influenza. It would be in the interest of humanity if doctors turned to this homoeopathic cure and obtained results which they do not appear to be able to achieve with orthodox drugs. (See also under Bathing).

INGROWING TOE NAIL

A 'V'-shaped notch may be cut in the centre of the tip of the nail, and a groove made down the centre with a nail file. Some find that filing the nail straight — level with the end of the toe — a better way.

Thickened nails should be filed carefully over the whole of the thickened portion to keep them thin, so that all cutting is made easy. By doing this there is also less pressure on the toe from footwear. This is most effective.

Keep the nail moist with Olive oil; or, get homoeopathic tincture of Hydrastis and carefully pack a wisp of cotton wool that has been soaked in the Hydrastis under the ingrowing portion. Use the tips of small tweezers for the purpose. Renew, morning and night.

A slice of Lemon tied over the nail, and kept on all night, will gradually soften the offender, so that it can be eased out of the flesh and cut as desired. (See also Nails).

Homoeopathic Magnetis Polus Australis has cured many cases, although it does not always act. Try the 30th. potency: five pills morning and night for two weeks.

INSECT BITES

Oil of Eucalyptus, oil of Thyme or distilled extract of Witch Hazel are all satisfactory for application. If homoeopathic mother tincture of Ledum is at hand, use that. For the effects of bites take Ledum 3. Five pills three times daily. Urtica urens 3 or Apis 3 are also fine remedies. Other satisfactory applications are Lemon juice or a cut Onion.

For collapse after a bite or a sting Homoeopathic Apis 30 or 200 will prove effective. Take a dose of three or four pills as soon after the sting as possible, and repeat the dose every ten minutes until four doses have been taken. This remedy also deals with collapse following bites and stings. Urtica urens taken in the same manner will also deal with this condition.

INSOMNIA

A really Hot Foot Bath, following by some deep Breathing exercises (see **Breathing**) will cure some cases of Insomnia, and help in all cases.

One reason for sleeplessness is the fear of not being able to sleep. This anxiety keeps the mind awake and the system tensed up. (See **Relaxation**). More often than not, it is psychological causes that keep sleep away. A happy mind, free from morbid thoughts, invites restful sleep. Should the sufferer have worries and troubles, it will be necessary to read what has been said on **Spiritual** Aid and **Psychology**.

Here is a very fine herbal remedy which helps to induce sleep without deadening the nerves:

Hops	½ ounce
Scullcap	1 ounce
Passion Flowers	½ ounce

Simmer in two pints of water, in an iron or enamel pot, for twenty minutes. Strain. Take a wineglassful before meals and another on retiring. The nightly dose should be taken warm for preference. If this fails, try the fresh plant tincture (obtainable from homoeopathic chemists) of Passion Flower (Passiflora); five or six drops in a little tepid water on retiring.

The idea of getting to sleep by 'counting sheep' is a waste of time in most cases. One successful method is to look at some small object in the room, or a small patch of light on the wall. Your eyes will soon tire if you look at the object open-eyed. Renew the effort, and soon the eyes will close in sleep. Probably the best way of all is to relax by means of the Eeman method, as discussed under **Relaxation**.

Another very successful method which can be employed when relaxing by the Eeman method, or when just remaining comfortable, is to review the events of the day *backwards*. Think backwards step by step from the moment of getting into bed. You may fall asleep before 'tea time'!

A slice of raw onion before retiring will act well with some people.

IPECACUANHA

Material doses produce vomiting; so homoeopathic doses cure vomiting, except in those cases where special causes exist. Ipecac. 3. is a fine remedy for coughs, bronchitis and vomiting. Also useful for leucorrhoea, as it tones the membranes of the female organs. The dose for the 3rd. potency is four or five pills three or four times daily. For the 30th. potency, a dose morning and night.

IRISH MOSS

This remedy is soothing and nourishing, supplying both food and medicine. Of great value in chronic respiratory troubles of every kind; also good for irritation of the kidneys and bladder, may be added to any herbal tea, or taken on its own. Steep half an ounce in cold water for ten minutes, then boil in three parts of water or milk, or in equal parts of water and milk, for fifteen minutes. Strain through linen and season with Honey, Liquorice, Cinnamon, Nutmeg, Lemon or any likeable flavouring to taste. Take a large cupful three times daily. Makes a good night-cap.

IRRITATION (Pruritus)

The cause may be acidity, blood disorganisation, pancreatic trouble etc., or the use of soaps containing soda and by some detergents. Sufferers should not use soda bath salts.

The medicine advised for **Auto-toxaemia** will help when the blood is out of order. (See also remarks under **Acidity**).

Sulphur ointment will help in some cases but it should not be used for long periods.

Balsaam of Peru may be gently massaged in at bedtime; oil of cade is also useful.

An excellent lotion can be made by mixing two ounces of glycerine with two of spirits of camphor, adding one heaped teaspoonful of borax and then heating slightly and shaking the bottle until the borax is dissolved. Apply two or three times daily.

Oil of lavender is very effective in some cases.

Homoeopathic remedies are Radium Bromide 30, five pills nightly for two weeks. Another effective remedy is Sulphur 3, five pills a few minutes before meals three times daily. Kreosotum 3 taken in the same manner as Sulphur has proved successful in many cases.

Itching of the anus may be due to worms, in which case it should be treated accordingly.

JABORANDI

Half to one teaspoonful of tincture of Jaborandi will cause profuse perspiration; hence it is useful as an eliminative medicine in colds and chest troubles. Large doses cause profuse salivation, the saliva pouring out of the mouth. Swelling of the parotid glands also takes place. From this we deduce that minute doses of Jaborandi are good for excessive sweating and mumps. For mumps take five pills of Jaborandi 3. every three hours: or, five pills of the 30th. potency morning and night. It is a most effective medicine.

Jaborandi 30. is also very useful in nervous disorders associated with a lack of co-ordination, black-outs, etc.

In material form it is an important ingredient in hair and scalp lotions. Taken internally in homoeopathic potency it encourages the growth of new hair.

JAUNDICE

Take ten drops of the fluid extract of Barberry (Berberis) in a little hot water three times daily. More effective remedies are homoeopathic Chelidonum 1 and Berberis 1. Take the Chelidonium before meals and the Berberis after meals for one to two weeks. Five pills to a dose. This clears the liver and gall bladder and tones up those organs.

JEALOUSY

'Jealousy is as cruel as the grave', so goes an old saying. Jealousy is a form of fear — fear of a rival. To be consumed with this negative emotion produces great debility and terrible unhappiness. Compassion is the cure. See what has been written under **Spiritual Aid** and **Psychology**. A useful medicine which has helped thousands of sufferers is homoeopathic Lachesis. Five pills of Lachesis 30. morning and night may be tried; but, as a rule, the 200th potency is more effective. Take five pills of Lachesis 200. on rising, again on retiring and a final dose on rising the next morning.

JOINTS

For stiffness of the joints, when not due to any actual disease, massage them with equal parts of warm Olive and Castor oil. Fomenting with a solution of a tablespoonful of Epsom salts in a bowl of hot water, is also helpful. Internally, take five pills of homoeopathic Bryonia 3. before meals, and five of Euphorbium 3. after meals.

JUNIPER BERRIES

An old remedy for indigestion and kidney disorders, and very effective it is. More recently, Juniper berries have been found effective for catarrh and weakness of the intestinal muscle.

Simmer one ounce of the berries in a pint of water for fifteen minutes. Dose: a small wineglassful before meals.

KELP (See Bladderwrack)

KIDNEY DISORDERS

The herbal medicine given under **Bladder** is also suitable for poor kidney function and weakness. See also **Runner Beans**.

There are several homoeopathic remedies, and their selection depends on the symptoms peculiar to each case. If a sufferer has kidney trouble which will not respond to the herbal tea, he should consult a homoeopathic repertory, or visit a reliable practitioner. In many cases Terebinth 3., five pills before meals, and Berberis Vulg. 3., five pills after meals, three times daily, will produce results. In others Gelsemium 3. and Drosera 3., taken in the same manner, are more suitable remedies. Other repertory remedies are: Belladonna, Erigeron, Lycopodium, Formica, Cantharis, Eupatorium Pur.

One excellent remedy, not usually given in repertories, but which will often act when all others fail, is Erbium 30. Five pills morning and night. All these remedies are harmless.

KOLA

An African native remedy used to stimulate the nerves. It also aids the heart. The action is probably due to the Caffeine content. Kola is taken by coloured people to enable them to undergo tasks requiring expenditure of energy. It is good for diarrhoea, and is said to lessen the craving for alcohol. The dose is ten to twenty drops in a little hot water before meals. Kola enters into many herbal tonics for giving strength and stamina.

LABRADOR TEA

Labrador Tea, or Marsh Tea (Ledum) is used as a tea in the usual infusion of one ounce to one pint of water, taken in small wineglassful doses, for colds, coughs and respiratory troubles generally. Ledum, used homoeopathically, is a good example of the wide range of uses that are covered when a simple remedy has been potentised. In homoeopathic form, Ledum becomes a fine remedy in cases of rheumatism, skin eruptions with irritation, marked coldness with fatigue and for wounds caused by sharp instruments. Of recent years, Ledum has been found to have a profound action on the suprarenal glands. These glands produce the 'energy hormone', and this explains why Ledum, given in minute doses, builds up the vital force. Another remedy with a somewhat similar action on the suprarenals is Agnus Castus. Agnus was, and still is, regarded as one of the outstanding remedies for debility caused by sexual abuses; it probably acts more upon the suprarenal glands than upon the generatives. Ledum is also a tonic to the eye lens.

For any of the complaints named, four or five pills of Ledum 3. before meals, will undoubtedly be of value; although we prefer the 30th. potency: a dose morning and night. The dosage for Agnus is the same.

LADIES SLIPPER

This plant is the Cypripedium of America. Half a teaspoonful of the fluid extract in hot water before meals is a good medicine for nervous disorders, neurasthenia, neuralgia, nervous headaches and female weakness. Given homoeopathically, in the 2x or 3x dilution, it is a wonderful remedy for teething children, insomnia (especially in the very young) and tummy troubles. It seems to act on the more placid mentality, while Chamomilla is the remedy for infants with irritable dispositions.

LARYNGITIS

In the early stages give five pills of Spongia 3. and five of Belladonna 3. every two hours in alternation. As the symptoms improve cease the Belladonna and take Hydrastis 3. instead. Cold throat packs will be helpful. Mix equal parts of Vinegar and cold water, soak a large handkerchief in this and apply loosely round the throat. Renew every hour at first, and later every six hours. (See also **Sore Throat**).

LAVENDER

Lavender tea is a gentle stimulant to the stomach and is helpful to the nerves. It modifies the harsh action of bitter stomach and bowel medicines when added to them. Some sufferers from nervous dyspepsia have found it to be very helpful indeed. A heaped teaspoonful of the flowers is placed in a jug with one pint of hot (not boiling) water. After half an hour it is ready for use. Take a tablespoonful before meals.

LAWS OF CORRESPONDENCE

As the Laws of Correspondence are linked with the old herbal Doctrine of Signatures, we shall discuss them jointly as being one and the same. The ancient herbalists believed that God has set a signature on plants so that human beings would know how to use them as medicine from their colour, appearance and structure. This may sound very much like 'an old wives tale'. The remarkable fact is that it is true!

Take, for example, the colour of flowers as being indications. Plants with yellow flowers were regarded as being useful for 'yellow complaints'. That is, ailments such as jaundice, yellow fever and disorders of the (yellow) bile. Thus, plants with yellow flowers should be good for indigestion, liver trouble, fevers associated with 'liverishness', gall disorders and bowel complaints. The Dandelion, Chelidonium and Berberis, to mention only three of a very large number, bear yellow blossoms, and all are regarded as outstanding remedies for these ailments. Furthermore, analysis reveals that they are rich in the mineral salts that activate the organs affected. Blue is a sedative colour, so it should be good for the nerves. Plants bearing blue flowers are nervines and sedatives, examples being Scullcap, Vervain, Valerain, etc. These plants are rich in natural phosphates so badly called for in nervous disorders. Red is stimulating; the colour suggests the blood. Plants bearing red flowers or red fruit are good for the blood, heart and circulation. The ripe, red Hawthorn berry, the Scarlet Pimpernel and the Red Clover are examples.

One must remember, of course, that trouble in one part or system in the human organism may be due entirely to a basic cause in another part or system; so it does not always follow that plants with red flowers will cure, say, a blood disorder affecting the skin, when the basic cause may be in the nervous system. As with all things accurate diagnosis and the discovery of the basic cause is necessary.

The same applies to shape and appearance. Old herbalists decided that the Scullcap, being shaped like a human skull, would be good for complaints in the head. It is so. The leaves of St. John's Wort suggested the lungs, and the red dots in the leaves suggested bleeding. Hence, they gave that remedy for lung complaints, haemorrhages, wounds, etc. We have no better remedy in these scientific days for such conditions. The roots of the Couch Grass look exactly like the urinary passages and the fallopian tubes. Few remedies can equal this plant for disorders of these passages. That is how the Doctrine of Signatures and the Laws of Correspondence had their genesis; and even today, we learn a great deal about the remedial value of plants from their colour and appearance.

The leaves of the Male Fern suggest the tape worm. This plant is one of the best ever discovered for expelling the parasite. Scores of examples could be mentioned, but those already discussed will serve to show how nature has symbolized in plants the uses to which they may be placed. One modern school of medicine, using homoeopathic type remedies, pays considerable attention to this ancient idea.

It is interesting to note how one part or organ of the body

has a corresponding relationship with another. The intestines are, in appearance, like an enlarged brain. The function of both is to absorb: the brain absorbs mental food; the intestines absorb physical nourishment. Disturbances in the one will affect the other. Many intestinal troubles may be traced to the mental assimilation of wrong ideas, or the refusal to absorb good thoughts. Lack of mental vigour, anxiety states and mental unbalance can cause intestinal trouble, and disorders of the intestines can also produce the same mental states. The colon (large intestine) is mainly an eliminative organ, and faulty elimination causes toxic states and many diseases. On the mental side the refusal to eliminate 'waste thoughts', morbidity and negative emotions will upset the physical colon. Proper treatment of the colon will aid the eliminative processes of the mind.

The heart is symbolic of love and courage, and it has been found that many psychological states of unfulfilled love, 'love sickness', jealousy, etc., will so upset the physical heart as to cause heart disease. On the other hand physical heart trouble undoubtedly tends to produce anxiety states in the mind.

The bladder eliminates waste in liquid form, and there is a correspondence between this and certain mental conditions. The same with the kidneys. The spleen, pancreas and other organs also have their mental correspondencies. Everybody knows how miserable a 'liverish' person can be. A morbid, nasty state of mind will upset the liver; likewise, a sick liver will upset the mind. The lungs are the 'leaves' of the human tree through which we draw in life. Lung disorders and shallow breathing lessen vitality of both mind and body. When we fail to expand our mental lungs and refuse to be receptive to the psychological breath of life we suffer in a similar manner. See also **Zone Therapy**, a science of healing closely associated with these laws.

LEMON

The Lemon is a refreshing tonic and cleanser of the system. It is useful in colds, fevers, indigestion, sluggish liver, toxic states, high blood pressure, arterial weakness and for external application. Indeed, lemonade may be spelt lemon-aid!

Those who find fresh lemons rather harsh to take may

roast them. For some people they are even better medicinally taken this way. Roast a lemon until it begins to crack open. Take a teaspoonful of the juice with a little Honey every hour for colds, coughs, sore throat and bronchitis.

Raw lemon juice will often abort a bilious attack. It is more potent for this purpose when a small eggspoonful of common table salt is well mixed with the juice of two lemons. Take a teaspoonful every few minutes until symptoms have cleared.

It is wise to use fresh lemons, or tinned lemon juice which is free from chemical preservatives. Lemon is also good for facial blemishes, freckles and chapped hands when applied locally. Lemon juice is frequently mentioned in this book for various purposes.

LEUCORRHOEA

Fluid extract of Golden Seal	1 ounce
Fluid extract of Echinacea	1 ounce
Tincture of Myrrh	1 ounce
Tincture of Ipecacuanha	1 teaspoonful

Dose: half a teaspoonful in a little hot water before meals three times daily. For those who prefer homoeopathic medicine four or five pills of Hydrastis 3. should be taken before meals, and the same of Ipecac. 3. after meals, three times daily.

Vaginal injections are also most helpful in severe cases. To two pints of warm water (blood heat) add a heaping teaspoonful of powdered Borax and about ten drops of fluid extract of Golden Seal (Hydrastis). Stir thoroughly. Inject this every morning for twenty-one days. Leucorrhoea is a result of poor health, a toxic state and/or over-indulgence in sex. Masturbation is also a cause. Moderation in the sex life and common sense is called for. The general health must be built up.

Leucorrhoea should never be suppressed with drugs, as such treatment can have serious consequences. If professional aid is necessary visit a reliable homoeopath, herbalist or nature cure practitioner.

There are many fine homoeopathic remedies, including Hydrastis, Kali Bic., Pulsatilla, Sepia and Thuja. Our own experience has led us to prescribe mostly remedies that are a little out of the ordinary. These are Ipecac., Bufo and Dirca. With these remedies in the 30th. potency we have had excellent results. The sufferer may either select a remedy according to the homoeopathic repertory or materia medica; or, try one of the three we prefer: four or five pills morning and night for a while. Should one fail, try another. Or, use one of the other homoeopathic remedies in the 30th. potency in the same manner.

LILY OF THE VALLEY

A harmless heart tonic and normaliser; said to be as good as Digitalis and possessing no harmful effects. It also aids the kidneys. Lily of the Valley (Convallaria) is good for valvular deficiency and dropsy. Ten drops of the fluid extract may be taken in a little warm water before meals with the knowledge that harm cannot result. Or, take Convallaria in homoeopathic form: four or five pills of the 3rd. potency before meals, three times daily.

LIME FLOWERS

A common domestic remedy for indigestion, headaches, hysteria and nervous disorders. Said to be useful for insomnia and catarrh. Brew one teaspoonful of the flowers in a teapot, as one would ordinary tea. Take a small cupful, warm, before or after meals. The flowers may be blended with ordinary tea and used as a beverage daily.

LINSEED

A valuable old remedy for colds, coughs, catarrh, bronchitis and inflamed states of the stomach and intestines. Has often proved effective in respiratory troubles when other medicines have failed. Simmer a tablespoonful of the seeds in a pint of water for ten minutes. Strain. Add Lemon and Honey to taste, and take a tablespoonful (warm for preference) every hour or two hours. May be added to other respiratory medicines and herbal teas. The crushed seeds make a valuable poultice for the chest in cases of bronchitis and congestion of the lungs. Just a very few people cannot take Linseed tea, but they are few. Linseed oil is good for cooking.

LIPS (CRACKED)

Take two tablets of Nat. Mur. 6x before meals, and two of Calc. Fluor. 6x after meals, three times daily. Also two tablets of Silica 12x first thing on rising and again on retiring. Or, try Flouric Acid 3. five pills before meals. Locally, anoint the lips two or three times daily with glycerine in which a few tablets of powdered Nat. Mur. 6x have been well mixed. Chickweed, Hydrastis or Marigold ointments are also helpful. The two latter should be obtained from homoeopathic chemists.

One of the best applications consists of twenty drops each of the mother tinctures, or fluid extracts, of Golden Seal and Marigold well shaken in half an ounce of glycerine. Apply two or three times daily.

LIQUORICE

The fluid extract, or the medicinal stick Liquorice, is often added to bitter medicine to cover the taste. Liquorice is good for coughs, bronchitis and asthma; also has some value for stomach acidity and constipation, as it is gently laxative. Pontefract cakes (sweets) will act as a laxative for children. Here is a grand old remedy for coughs and bronchitis: one ounce of Liquorice root, a teaspoonful of Linseed and a good handful of best Raisins. Place in two quarts of soft water and simmer gently for about an hour. Then add four tablespoonsful of best Honey and a good tablespoonful of Lemon juice. Mix thoroughly.

Take a dessertspoonful to a tablespoonful whenever the cough is troublesome, and a cupful when going to bed. It is better taken warm. Do not prepare this remedy in an aluminium pot.

LIVER TROUBLE

A bad liver causes the sufferer to become morbid, and even nasty-minded. In these cases attention to diet is essential.

Five to ten drops of the fluid extract of Berberis (Barberry) is an effective medicine in many cases. Take in hot water before meals. Lemon and Salt is also helpful (see under Lemon). For obstinate, deeply-seated liver troubles, homoeopathic remedies are the best. Two very outstanding medicines are Opium 30. and Podophyllum 30. Take five pills of Opium

30. on rising, and five of Podophyllum 30. on retiring, for two or three weeks. In cases where there is a pain under the lower part of the right shoulder-blade, take five pills of Chelidonium 3. before meals. In 'nervy' cases with a sluggish liver, Hydrastis 3. (5 pills) should be tried before meals; or, five pills of Hydrastis 30. morning and night.

When the above remedies fail, and the gall bladder is involved, try five pills of Cholesterin 30. morning and night.

Sufferers should avoid cooked animal fats and fried foods.

LOBELIA

There are several Lobelias, the best known being Lobelia Inflata. The famous herbalist, Dr. Samuel Thompson, made a great reputation for himself by using Lobelia as an emetic in a vast number of disorders; his idea being that by clearing out foul matter from the stomach, and relaxing the system, nature would do all that was necessary for recovery. An enormous amount of good has been accomplished using Lobelia in this manner. It is not a poison, but its use by inexperienced people may produce rather frightening symptoms. In minute doses there can be no alarming effects whatever. Lobelia is grand for coughs and respiratory troubles, Asthma, etc. Take three drops of the fluid extract in hot, sweetened water every three hours. Each dose acts better if one or two drops of tincture of Cayenne have been added.

We prefer Lobelia in homoeopathic potency, when it becomes a far more deeply-acting remedy. In potency it is not only excellent for asthma and lung troubles, but is one of the finest of remedies for nervous and intestinal disorders, and those conditions where the system is tensed up. For indigestion, 'nerviness', coughs, bronchitis, bowel indigestion, flatulence and abdominal pain take five pills of Lobelia 3. every two hours, and then less frequently. Even better results follow the taking of a dose of the 30th. potency morning and night for a time.

The herbal acid tincture of Lobelia is also good for these troubles. It is more suitable in most cases than the fluid extract and, unless taken in large doses, does not cause vomiting. The dose for the acid tincture is five to ten drops in water before meals for any of the complaints mentioned.

Cayenne may be added. Use small doses for children.

LOCKJAW

Give the sufferer a hot foot bath and call professional aid. Helpful medicines to take are Aconitum 3., five pills every hour. Aconitum is the remedy when the trouble has been caused by cold. When it is due to injuries take Hypericum 1x in dilution: five drops in a teaspoonful of hot water every hour. Homoeopathic Mephites 30. is regarded by some practitioners as being a specific. Take five pills every hour for six hours, and then a dose morning and night. Another good remedy is Opium 30., dose the same as for Mephites.

LOVE

True love is a great force which in its highest form brings about mental and physical well-being but this perfect expression of selflessness is seldom found to-day.

Few people know what true love is; fewere still attempt to put it into practice.

Selfish love has nothing to do with the perfect form of love which is selflessness, kindness, compassion, tolerance, generosity without the thought of self.

He who understands love in its highest form has found peace and contentment.

Love is complete and total service *without thought of self* and anyone attempting to tread this path is on the road to heaven.

Christ said 'I say unto you, love your enemies' and it is a fact that when we love our enemies we cease to have any! The late Professor Drummond wrote a beautiful discourse on love entitled 'The Greatest Thing in the World' which is recommended to every reader of this book.

If you make love a ruling incentive throughout life by thinking of others and helping with their problems, you will find that you feel better yourself!

LUMBAGO

When the pain is increased by movement, give 5 pills of Bryonia 3. every two hours. When movement tends to relieve, give Rhus Tox. 3. 5 pills, a dose every two hours. A Bran poultice to the small of the back is helpful. The treatment given for **Rheumatism** is very effective.

LUNG WEAKNESS

The medicines given under **Bronchitis** and **Coughs** are most useful, and will strengthen the organs of respiration.

We suggest the following be tried by those who are troubled by continual coughing and mucous expectoration; five pills of homoeopathic Calcarea Carb. 30 on rising, and five of Lycopus Virg. 30 on retiring for three or four weeks. Then give the remedies a rest for a week or so. If there is improvement, but the trouble has not totally cleared, take a follow-up course of the remedies.

Slippery Elm and Irish Moss are both excellent lung food remedies and may be taken with advantage by all sufferers in addition to other remedies.

MALARIA

Cut Peruvian bark	½ ounce
Bonset	½ ounce
Scullcap	½ ounce
Yarrow	½ ounce

Simmer in two pints of water in an iron or enamel pot for twenty minutes. Strain. Give a tablespoonful every hour. As the patient improves administer less frequently. This medicine is excellent for this trouble. Give the patient all the hot lemon he desires.

For those who prefer homoeopathic medicine give five pills of Millifolium 30. in alternation with five of Anacardium 30. every hour. That is: a dose of Millifolium at 8 a.m., one of Anacardium at 9 a.m., Millifolium at 10 a.m., and so on. As symptoms improve give alternately every two hours. Or, give the Millifolium 30. in alternation with China Sulph. 30. in the same manner. As a rule very nervy people respond better to Anacardium.

MALE FERN

Male Fern (Filix Mas.) is used in material doses for the expulsion of tape worm. At night take two or three teaspoonsful of the fluid extract in a little hot water, with Lemon juice added. Half an hour later take a dose of Castor oil. May be repeated in two or three days time if not successful.

Herbalists have used Male Fern as a worm remedy for a

very long time. Homoeopaths have discovered fairly recently that when this plant is potentised it becomes a powerful medicine for weak hearts and varicose veins. It somewhat resembles Digitalis in its action on the heart, without any of the harmful effects of the latter. It is also good for an irritable colon. Take four or five pills of Filix Mas. 30. on rising and on retiring, for two or three weeks. The heart condition calling for Filix Mas. has a bounding, irregular pulse.

MALIGNANCY

In all cases of malignancy, or suspected malignancy, seek immediate professional advice. Right thinking and living should ensure that one does not fall a victim to these disorders, and we stress that good thought is not enough, and that living to the rules is not enough — both are essential. Fear of malignancy can produce that which is feared in course of time, and many cancers have been due to fear alone. It is against the present laws for us to suggest any actual treatment. We deplore the fact that money supplied by good-intentioned people for cancer research is used in searching for a virus which is only a result of deeper causes.

MALNUTRITION

The general health must be improved. See under Diet, Bathing, Breathing, Exercise. The medicine advised for Anaemia will be most beneficial. The thorough mastication of all food is essential, and we have known this to be all that was necessary in some cases.

An eggspoonful of plain extract of malt in a tumbler of hot water, milk and water, or milk, taken in sips two or three times daily before meals, has been of service in a vast number of cases. An eggspoonful of the malt is ample — too much is not so satisfactory. Those with weak livers should take the malt in more water than milk; or, in water only. (See also under Indigestion).

MANDRAKE (AMERICAN)

One of the finest liver tonics, and a purgative in material doses. The dose for purgative effects if five to thirty drops in water. Some people require a smaller dose than others.

Employed homoeopathically, it not only activates the liver (it is a liver 'builder' and gives tone to the organ) but does much to restore a sluggish or defective liver to health. Liver sufferers should take five pills of Mandrake (Podophyllum) 30. on rising and on retiring. Cease the remedy when feeling really better.

MARIGOLD

Marigold (Calendula) tea is good for feverish conditions and measles. It also raises the resistance to colds. Place an ounce of the petals in a jug, pour on a pint of boiling water and allow to stand for half an hour. Strain. The dose varies according to age. Two or three teaspoonsful are enough for the very young, while adults may take a wineglassful, three times daily. Marigold is an ingredient in many reliable ointments for wounds, varicose veins and ulcers. Very fine for skin disorders. The Marigold is one of the best healers of wounds ever discovered, and the tincture was used for the wounds of soldiers during the two world wars. A few drops added to a wineglass of cold water make an excellent dressing for any injury. The petals, moistened with warm water, also form an excellent local application. Marigold ointment, as made by homoeopathic chemists, is recommended. Calendula 3., five pills three times daily, is good taken internally for the effects of injuries, ulcers and vein troubles.

MARJORAM (WILD)

Used as a tea to promote the monthly period, and as a general stimulant. In homoeopathy it is one of the best remedies for female troubles. For disorders of the uterus it is very effective, and appears to have an affinity with that organ. It also strengthens the eyes and improves the sight. In both sexes it is a fine remedy for the effects of sexual abuse. We recommend the 30th. potency. Marjoram is known as Origanum Vulg. Take four or five pills morning and night.

MARRIAGE

A section on marriage is included in this work because it can have a profound effect on health and happiness.

Many physical symptoms originate in the mind and a

happy marriage can create harmony and thus make an important contribution to well-being.

The ideal state is where the partners attain a good degree of harmony on the physical, spiritual and intellectual planes.

There should be mutual respect and the partners should endeavour to avoid over indulgence in sex which often leads to unhappiness, especially where one of the partners feels a reluctance to participate. It is impossible to suggest what is normal in sexual activity as we all differ in our needs but it must be emphasized that everyone should try to be considerate in making demands in this field.

MARSHMALLOW

A popular old remedy for bronchitis, coughs and complains of the urinary organs when inflamed and painful states are present. The crushed or powdered roots also make an excellent poultice. Like Slippery Elm, it is as potent for external healing as it is for internal purposes.

The powdered root may be mixed with Slippery Elm powder to make a soothing, healing and nourishing food-remedy. Use a teaspoonful of the combined powders as a dose. Mix with Honey or brown sugar and make into a paste with a little cold water. Then add hot milk, stirring briskly. An infusion of the leaves is taken frequently in wineglassful doses for respiratory and urinary troubles. Place an ounce of the leaves in a jug; pour on a pint of boiling water and allow to stand for thirty minutes. Strain. It is usually taken warm.

MASSAGE

Massage for healing purposes goes back to the genesis of history. It is instinctive and natural to rub any part of the anatomy that has been hurt, or is painful. Hence, massage is good for many disorders associated with nerve and muscle pains: rheumatism, fibrositis, sciatica, etc. Olive oil may be used for massage, but the dry hands are usually better. Oil, however, is nourishing for weak bodies. The human hand is the chief instrument of the brain, and its intelligent use can do a great deal for suffering. Employed lightly (stroking) the hands are soothing, and a healthy person can give ease in nervous troubles by lightly stroking the affected areas. The hands of a normal person are a source of human magnetism, and this healing force can be transmitted to the sufferer. Indeed, many cures of nervous and other troubles have been achieved by making passes over the sufferer, but without actual contact. We have known a few passes from the front to the back of the head soothe an hysterical subject within two or three minutes.

Rheumatism, sciatica and painful congestions call for deep massage. The thumbs or fingers press deeply into the tissues, and the parts are kneeded with circular movements. The muscles are squeezed, morbid deposits are sent into the circulation for elimination, and a series of regular treatments can result in a cure, or great relief. However, *massage should never be applied over an inflamed area;* although magnetic passes may be used.

MAGNETIC TREATMENT

The sufferer is seated. The operator stands behind the patient and holds both hands with fingers extended three to six inches above and over the top-front of the head. The hands are moved backwards and downward over the back of the head and neck, each pass taking from one to two seconds. To return the hands to the top of the head the operator sweeps his hands outwards and away from the patient. The hands do not touch during the movements over the patient; they are held slightly apart. The treatment may be continued for five to ten minutes. Sometimes patients fall asleep during treatment, which is all to the good. This head treatment is good for mental tension, irritability, hysteria and insomnia.

In nervous cases head treatment may be followed by making passes down the whole length of the spine from the neck to the hips for a few minutes. This is excellent for nervous disorders. Treatment may be given daily, or two or three times weekly.

GENTLE MASSAGE

This is performed by stroking the affected areas lightly with the flat hands. While massage in any direction is good, the best effects are usually obtained by always stroking towards the heart. Stroking movements are sedative, and are employed to relieve nerve pains, neuralgia, aching in the muscles, etc. Sometimes somewhat better results are obtained if the pressure is slightly increased. Treatments should be given for five to ten minutes, depending on circumstances, and should take place daily, or two or three times weekly. The more the patient can relax during treatment, the better the effects.

KNEADING

The muscles are kneaded to relieve deep pain in rheumatic conditions, painful joints (unless they are inflamed, when no massage should be given apart from very gentle stroking or magnetic passes), sciatica, etc. Thumbs or fingers may be used. As a rule the thumbs are better. Press into the tissues and move them with a circular motion, changing the locality slightly from time to time. For sciatica the main treatment should be applied to the lower part of the spine and the buttock on the affected side. Treatment is painful, but produces good results. Deep stroking may also be applied up the affected leg. It is good to conclude any deep kneading with a few stroking movements.

The spine may be treated in all nervous conditions. Spinal massage improves the local blood circulation, frees the vital nerves from congestion and aids the functional activity of organs supplied with nerve force from the spine. The thumbs are used with deep circular movements on either side of the spine (the patient should be face downwards). The tissues are moved outwards away from the spine. Start from the neck and gradually work downwards. To treat the neck the patient should be seated. Any tender area should be worked on thoroughly. Most people are tender at the base of the skull, and this very important locality should receive special attention.

Treating the spine will assist in the recovery of almost any ailment from nervous exhaustion to indigestion, poor circulation and bowel disorders. Keep it up! With practice most people can perform these simple massage treatments at home.

When treating joints work well round the part; but remember not to deal with any part that is inflamed. For example, do not massage the knee for synovitis, but deep massage *under* the knee will be helpful.

In professional practice there are other forms of massage, but the simple methods we have considered in brief cover what is necessary for use in the home. (See also **Zone Therapy**).

MEADOWSWEET

This common wayside plant has been used by herbalists for generations as a remedy for urinary weakness and the diarrhoea of children. It is also a fine remedy for acidity. It is undoubtedly a good general tonic, and, as it is rich in Silica, it should have a wider range of action than is generally thought. According to the homoeopaths, Meadowsweet is indicated for those who are morbidly conscientious – the very 'faddy'. The infusion of one ounce in a pint of water is taken in small wineglassful doses before meals. This is an excellent remedy to try when one is 'out of sorts'.

MEASLES

Marigold tea is a very good remedy; or get half an ounce each of Bonset herb, Scullcap and Marigold. Simmer for fifteen minutes in a pint of water. Strain. Sweeten. Give a teaspoonful to a tablespoonful, according to age, every two hours.

The biochemic treatment consists of two tablets of Ferr. Phos. 6x and two of Kali Mur. 6x taken alternately every hour until better, and then less frequently. Homoeopathic Belladonna 3. is also excellent. Give five pills with each dose of Ferr. Phos. Do not combine the herbal with the homoeopathic treatment; use one or the other.

Keep the sufferer in a warm but airy room. Sponge down occasionally with Vinegar, or equal parts of Vinegar and water.

MELILOTUS

Melilotus, or King's Clover, is one of the best remedies for headaches, whether congestive or due to indigestion. In order to obtain the best effects the fresh plant tincture should be employed, as ordinary tinctures and extracts lose most of their curative value in the making.

May be taken for sick headache, throbbing headache, nervous headache, 'nerviness', indigestion, nerve pains and flatulence. Often very effective for nose-bleed. The dose is three to five drops in a teaspoonful of warm water every fifteen minutes until better. May also be used for inhaling, for which purpose put a few drops in a small jug of hot water; hold the face over the jug and cover the head with a towel to keep in the fumes. Inhale deeply. Can be obtained from all homoeopathic chemists.

MENOPAUSE

There are several outstanding homoeopathic remedies to help at this time of life. The mental symptoms may be taken as a guide to remedy selection. For example, some women are very jealous at this season of their lives, so Lachesis 30. (a dose morning and night) will be very helpful. Sepia is more suitable for others who are suspicious and inclined to shyness. Caulophyllum is a good all-round remedy for many of the physical symptoms. The 30th. potency is advised morning and night. All three of the remedies named assist in relieving the distressing flushes, although Dr. Guyon Richards recommends either Tantalum 30. or Fuchsia 30.

American Indian women take Blue Cohosh. This is the Caulophyllum of the homoeopaths. In fluid extract form it is highly recommended by the herbal school. If taken in this form the dose is ten to twenty drops in a little warm water before meals.

MENSTRUAL DISORDERS

For painful and obstructed menstruation this old herbal tea is strongly recommended:

Pennyroyal	½ ounce
Tansy	½ ounce

Simmer in one pint of water for fifteen minutes, using an iron or enamel pot. Take a wineglassful, hot, every three hours. Cease when the menses appear. The medicine is improved by adding two drops (not more) of Pulsatilla tincture to each dose taken. If the two herbs are taken in fluid extract form the dose is half a teaspoonful of each together in hot water. The tea acts better in most cases. Must not be taken by pregnant females. To strengthen the reproductive organs and help to normalize function, take the following medicine between periods:

| Motherwort | ½ ounce |
| Raspberry leaves | ½ ounce |

Prepare as for the Pennyroyal and Tansy combination, and take a wineglassful before meals, three times daily. If suffering from delayed or obstructed menses take the first mentioned medicine three days before the period is due.

The homoeopathic remedies advised under **Menopause** are also excellent for disorders of the reproductive system.

MENTAL REMEDIES

While morbid mental states call for psychological re-adjustment, many can be helped to an astonishing degree with homoeopathic remedies. We have known sufferers on the verge of insanity brought back to health by the employment of the correct homoeopathic remedy. Use the 30th. or the 200th. potency. Results can hardly be expected from the lower potencies and the best effects are obtained from the 200th. or higher. If the 30th potency is tried the suggested dose is three or four pills morning and night for two or three weeks. If taking a remedy in the 200th. potency take five pills on rising, five on retiring and five again on rising the next morning — three doses in all. These suggestions apply to each homoeopathic remedy mentioned.

All homoeopathic physicians recommend medicines for mental conditions, although those advised by the late Dr. Guyon Richards are, in our opinion, the best. The following remedies are mainly those according to Dr. Richards.

FEAR (General): Crotalus Hor.

ANXIETY: Plumbum.

ANXIETY FOR OTHERS: Platina.

APPREHENSION: Arnica.

CLAUSTROPHOBIA: Digitalis.

AGORAPHOBIA: Aconitum.

INFERIORITY: Silica, or Arsen. Alb.

ANXIETY OVER HUSBAND: Arnica.

DEPRESSION: Cadmium Sulph., or Elaps.

SHYNESS (Excessive): Sepia.

FAMILY WORRY: Hypericum.

SHOCK: Vanadium, Phos., or Arnica. For shock following abdominal operations Vanadium is the best remedy.

WORRY (General): Sepia.

FEAR OF BEING ALONE: Silica.

WORRY (Financial): Natrum Mur.

HEART (Psychological): Cactus Grand., or Anacardium.

FEAR CONCERNING STATE OF LUNGS: Argentum Nit.

FEARS WORSE AT NIGHT: Daphne.

FRIGHTENED TO GO TO SLEEP: Phytolacca.

LASSITUDE (usually with heart weakness): Jacaranda.

EMOTIONAL FEARS: Natrum Mur., or Aurum-Nat.-Mur.

JEALOUSY: Lachesis.

IMPATIENCE: Jaborandi (also known as Pilocarpus).

HURRY: Medorrhinum, or Psorinum.

SELF-PITY: Baptisia, or Selenium.

HUSTLE: Anacardium.

FIDGETINESS: Calc. Carb., or Epiphegus.

BRAIN OVER ACTIVE: Aconitum, or Kali Cyan.

DOMINATING DISPOSITION: Ignatia.

FUSSING OVER HEALTH: Mentha Pulegum.

POOR CONCENTRATION: Arsen. Alb., or Silica.

POOR WILL POWER: Cereus Serp., or Silica.

CONCEIT ABOUT APPEARANCE: Coca.

SUSPICION: Sepia, or Lachesis.

LACK OF FAITH: Pulsatilla.

LACK OF COURAGE: Silica, or Cadmium Sulph.

NON-POSITIVE: Arsen. Alb., or Silica.

DESPONDENCY: Mezereum, or Cadmium Sulph.

DREAD: Belladonna.

VACILLATING DISPOSITION: Staphisagria.

FUSSINESS (General): Lil. Tig.

FUDDLED HEAD: Hyoscyamus

TOUCHINESS (hair-trigger disposition): Calc. Carb., or Chamomilla.

MONGOLISM: Cerato.

FEELING OF BEING OVER-SHADOWED: Variolinum, or China Sulph.

INHIBITION: Platina, or Silica.

MENTAL LAZINESS: Aesculus Hip.

MENTAL SLUGGISHNESS — SLOW TO ACT: Mezereum.

POOR MEMORY: Rosemarinus, Staphisagria, or Anacardium.

FEAR OF CANCER: Crotalus Hor.

FEAR OF CRITICISM: Silica.

FEAR OF EVIL: Sepia.
HOPELESSNESS: Cadmium Sulph.
RESENTMENT: Cadmium Sulph.
LOVE OF WORK (Excessive): Argentum Nit.
LACK OF MENTAL COHESION: Kali Mur., or Silica.
DIFFICULT TO CONTROL THOUGHTS: Nat. Mur.
IRRITATED BY OTHERS: Ignatia, or Thallium Oxide.
IRRITABLE CHILDREN: Chamomilla.
FEARS DATING FROM INFANCY: Naja Trip.
FEARS OF FITS: Helonias.
FEAR OF PERSECUTION: Belladonna.
FEAR OF DEATH: Crotalus Hor., or Aconitum.
EMOTIONALISM: Nat. Mur., Aurum-Nat.-Mur., Equisetum, Sumbul.
FEAR OF THE SEA: Naja Trip.
FEAR OF BREAKDOWN: Silica.
CANNOT RELAX: Platina, Sumbul, Nat. Mur., or Equisetum.
FEAR OF SUICIDE: Cannabis Sat., or Silica. Kali Phos. also helpful.
FEAR OF EXMINATIONS: Silica.
FEAR OF LOSS OF MOTION: Agaricus.
FEAR OF INSANITY: Cannabis Sat.
LACK OF CONFIDENCE: Lycopodium, or Pulsatilla.
LACKING IN TRUSTFULNESS: Nat. Mur.
ANXIETY OVER CAREER: Aconitum, or Silica.
PITY FOR OTHERS CAUSING ILLNESS (excess pity): Bismuth.
OVER-SENSITIVE: Silica, Nat. Mur., or Anacardium.
ANXIETY OVER STATE OF STOMACH: Platina.
CRUELTY: Bufo, or Aloe.
AVERSION TO PHYSICAL LABOUR: Anacadium, or Rhododendron.
AVERSION TO MENTAL LABOUR: Aesculus Hip.
FEAR OF FAILURE: Helonias.
MELANCHOLIA: Helonias, Silica, Nat. Mur., or Anacardium.
DESPAIR: Cadmium Sulph., or Silica.
FEAR OF THUNDER: Rhododendron, and Silica.
MENTAL CONFUSION: Hyoscyamus, Anacardium, or Kali Mur. Pituitary 30. is also helpful in some cases.
VACANT MIND: Silica, Kali Phos., Anacardium, or Kali Cyan.

Another deservedly popular treatment for mental states is by means of the Bach remedies. These are not homoeopathic, but are akin in that the doses are minute. For details readers are referred to the books written by Dr. Bach on the subject. Here we give only a very brief reference to the remedies and their uses.

ROCK ROSE: Terror.
MIMULUS: Ordinary fears.
CHERRY PLUM: Great fear and fear of death.
ASPEN: Fear of the unknown. Most useful for the fears of children.
RED CHESTNUT: Anxiety for others.
CERATO: Lack of confidence in one's intuition.
SCLERANTHUS: Indecision.
GENTIAN: Lack of faith in the self.
GORSE: Total hopelessness and despair.
HORNBEAM: Results of over-work.
WILD-OAT: Frustration.
CLEMATIS: Indifference — a dreamy state.
HONEYSUCKLE: Living in the past.
WILD ROSE: Resignation. Giving up.
OLIVE: Psychic and mental exhaustion.
WHITE CHESTNUT: Any type of obsession.
MUSTARD: Depression due to unknown causes.
CHESTNUT BUD: Failure to learn from experience.
WATER VIOLET: Aloofness.
IMPATIENS: Impatience.
HEATHER: Self-love. Selfishness.
AGRIMONY: For those who prefer to suffer in silence.
CENTAURY: Undue and unwise 'giving' to others.
WALNUT: For those in need of protection from others, and from the affairs of life.
HOLLY: Jealousy. For nasty mental states.
LARCH: For a feeling of inferiority.
PINE: Self-condemnation.
ELM: Excess of ambition and enthusiasm.
SWEET CHESTNUT: Intense anxiety.
STAR OF BETHLEHEM: Shock. (Especially when digestion is upset).
WILLOW: Always blaming others.

OAK: For those who have to struggle through life.

CRAB APPLE: For clearing the mind and body of poisonous thoughts and their effects.

CHICORY: General fussiness.

VERVAIN: Mental and nervous strain.

VINE: Excess of self-confidence.

BEECH: Intolerance.

ROCK WATER: For self-martyrs.

Here is a combination of Bach remedies which makes a most valuable medicine for shock, fear, sudden illness, accidents and all cases of emergency. It has been called 'The rescue remedy'. Take a one ounce bottle and half fill it with fresh water, or distilled water. Then add one or two drops of Rock Rose, Clematis, Impatiens, Star of Bethlehem and Cherry Plum. Fill up the bottle with brandy (to act as a preservative). The dose is two or three drops in a little water. Repeat in a few minutes, and then every two or three hours while necessary.

Obtain the Dr. Bach remedies from homoeopathic chemists. The usual dose for any one remedy is a single drop in a little water, two or three times daily. If the mental symptoms call for more than one remedy the selected items may be taken together.

MENTHOL

Menthol applicators and ointments are very soothing when applied to the forehead and back of the neck for headaches. A little Menthol ointment in each nostril aids breathing in catarrhal cases, and has some value in clearing up colds. For coughs and bronchitis, apply cloths wrung out in hot water to the chest and back; dry quickly and rub in Menthol ointment. There are several good brands on the market. Some rheumatic sufferers find this ointment good for painful joints and muscles.

MEZEREUM

This is the Spurge Olive, or Spurge Laurel. It is advised in homoeopathic form only, when it is a grand remedy for despondency and mental depression. Take five pills of Mezereum 30. morning and night, for two or three weeks. Or,

five pills of Mezereum 200. on rising, and again on retiring
for one day only, and await results.

MILK

A great deal has been written both for and against the use
of milk as a beverage. Some say that it is for calves and goats
only. These people are the strict vegetarians, and while their
arguments make some sense they do not make good sense in
this rather senseless world. At least one does not have to
slaughter an animal to obtain its milk, and well-kept cows
appear to be happy animals.

But, say some, a great deal of milk is T.B. infected; hence
unfit for human consumption. This brings up the question of
the germ theory. We doubt whether T.B. can be caused by
drinking milk in reasonably healthy people; or, indeed, in any
person.

Pasteurised milk elminates the germ danger (if it exists?);
but pasteurised milk is 'dead' milk, and is not by any means
the same food as fresh, clean milk. The applied heat not only
kills bacteria, but destroys much of the life-giving properties
of the milk. If afraid of germs, one can always purchase the
top grade T.B. tested, and use that.

We like to face facts, and the facts are that good milk is as
near to human blood in its chemical composition as any fluid
can be; thus it is a good food. It can and does build healthy
children, and will help to keep children and adults healthy.
Sick people are always helped by going on to baby foods; so
milk is an excellent food/remedy for invalids. In some nature
cure health homes patients are placed on an exclusive milk
diet for the treatment of all manner of disorders. All the
available evidence proves beyond question that most excellent results are thus obtained. The exclusive milk diet usually
follows a fast. The fast cleanses the system and prepares it to
receive the milk. On this diet from six to ten quarts of milk
may be taken daily, according to the decision of the
supervising practitioner. It is vital that the milk must be
masticated and not swallowed in gulps. Milk is a food, and all
foods must be 'chewed'. When a baby suckles, it performs a
chewing motion which causes the saliva to mix with the milk,
thus ensuring proper digestion. (See Diet). Milk should be
taken slowly and turned around in the mouth a few times

before swallowing. Some use a straw, which is of help.

The writer has brought health to several invalids, especially neurasthenics, by placing them on the exclusive milk diet. The milk may be taken for one to four weeks, and no other food. The greatest problem is constipation, which often takes place during the first few days. Prune juice every morning and evening will usually put this right; or, employ the enema occasionally.

A modified milk diet may be tried at home for all cases of malnutrition, debility, digestive disorders and nervous troubles. Take some prune juice first thing every morning followed by a tumbler of fresh milk half an hour later. Then take a tumbler of milk in sips, masticating every mouthful, every hour throughout the day. On retiring take more prune juice. If desired, at one or two periods during the day, take either a few dates or some fresh orange juice instead of the milk; or, at the same time.

Should the bowels become costive use an enema. If this is not possible take some Senna Pod tea. However, do not use a purgative unless it is essential. As a rule the prune juice will keep the bowels active.

It is wise to go without food for one day before commencing the milk diet, taking water or fruit juices only. After the milk cure the first meals should be very light, consisting of fruit or fresh salad only.

MISTLETOE

A fine old remedy for nervous disorders, spasms, high blood pressure and weak hearts. It is a harmless anti-spasmodic of great power. Sufferers should take ten to twenty drops of the fluid extract in a little hot water before meals, three times daily. Better results will follow the taking of the fresh plant tincture (from homoeopathic chemists), when the dose is five to ten drops in a little water before meals. Some outstanding cures have followed the taking of Mistletoe (Viscum Album), including valvular heart disease, high blood pressure, neurasthenia and arterial troubles. Mistletoe is a very useful medicine in some cases of rheumatism, especially when nervous symptoms are present.

MOLASSES

This is another of the 'cure-alls'. Don't believe it! Some people just cannot take Molasses — not even very small quantities. On the other hand, it is a fine remedy for constipation, mineral deficiency diseases and for some cases of rheumatism, always provided the sufferer can take it without upset. Half to one teaspoonful is dissolved in a tumbler of warm water and taken before breakfast, and again last thing at night. Costive people may soak prunes in water in which Molasses has been dissolved. Allow to soak over-night, and take with the prunes and some 'All-Bran' in the morning.

It is claimed by some writers that Molasses will help to prevent malignancy. This is probably true in some circumstances, as there are many valuable mineral salts in this substance which help to keep the blood chemically balanced. So, if you can take Molasses, have a little every day.

MONO-DIET

The mono-diet is a system of feeding on only one kind of food at a time. The idea is that this calls for less effort on the part of the digestive and assimilative organs. It is most helpful in cases of weakness of the digestive organs, malnutrition and general debility. Some writers claim pleasing results in the treatment of other ailments by adopting this system for a period of time. However, the food selected must be a complete food, otherwise the body is likely to be starved of protein, minerals or vitamins, etc. The exclusive Milk diet is an example of the ideal mono-method. (See Milk).

Some animals feed exclusively on one type of food. Take the Koala bear of Australia: this animal feeds and thrives on the leaves of the Eucalyptus tree, finding in these leaves all the materials necessary to maintain health and vitality. There is no doubt that civilised peoples take too many mixtures, and that such complex concoctions are a strain on the digestion, especially in the weakly. We recall a tired and rather faded lady who regained her vigour to a marked degree by eating nothing but compost grown flour in the form of stale wholemeal bread and porridge. She also practised thorough mastication. On no account should one try to live on white bread — the result would be disastrous, as white bread is not worthy of the name 'food', and to try to live on this and nothing else would result in disease.

One may try living for a week or two on whole grain products; although, in all cases, soaked prunes for breakfast would seem to be advisable to keep the bowels active. Some can live entirely on raw salads for long periods of time to the benefit of their minds and bodies. In our experience raw food without other body-building materials does not agree with all, and in no circumstances is it advised for more than a month at a time, except under expert supervision.

There is no doubt that even a week on a mono-diet will give the digestion a partial rest, and there are few people who will not benefit by trying this occasionally. On the exclusive Milk diet the period may be longer.

MORNING SICKNESS

Peach leaf tea (see **Peach**) will take away this trouble of pregnancy in many cases. Experience suggests that homoeopathic remedies are best. There are several of them: Ipecacuanha, Petroleum and Tabacum being examples. Try either. Take five pills of the selected remedy in the 30th. potency on rising and on retiring for as long as is necessary. Perhaps the most effective remedy of all, and one which we have never known to fail, is Actaea Racemosa in the 200th potency. Take five pills on rising, five on retiring and five again the following morning. Repeat in a week's time if necessary.

MOTHERWORT

This herb has been employed for generations as a soothing nerve tonic, and as a regulator of the female reproductive organs. It also has some positive value as a strengthener of the heart function. Many remedies are recommended for these disorders in this book, and any herb or medicine recommended may be tried with confidence. When one fails to produce the desired results another can be tried, without doing any harm. Motherwort tea should be considered as a reliable remedy for all female irregularities, painful periods, local inflammations, heart distress and 'nerviness'. Infuse one ounce of the leaves in one pint of boiling water, and allow to stand for an hour. Strain. Dose: a small wineglassful before meals three times daily.

MOUNTAIN ASH

How refreshingly invigorating to gaze on a Rowan tree (Mountain Ash) when it is laden with glossy red berries! Crush about one ounce of the ripe berries and place in a jug. Pour on one pint of hot water, and allow to stand for an hour. This makes an excellent gargle for sore throats, and also a fine vaginal injection for leucorrhoea. Such an injection may be given daily if necessary. The infusion is also good for diarrhoea, the dose being a tablespoonful every three hours. Children less according to age.

MOUNTAIN FLAX

This is regarded as being superior to Senna as a laxative. Acts on the bowels and kidneys, and certainly has some value in muscular rheumatism and catarrh, especially when associated with costiveness. Infuse one ounce of the herb in a pint of boiling water; allow to stand for an hour. Dose: a tablespoonful to a wineglassful, two or three times daily. Or, half a teaspoonful of the fluid extract in some hot water.

MOUNTAIN LAUREL

This is the Kalmia of the homoeopaths, and we advise it in homoeopathic form for weak hearts associated with violent palpitation and heart 'shocks'. Take four or five pills of the 3rd potency before meals, three times daily. In many instances better results will follow from the 30th. potency, when the dose should be five pills on rising and five on retiring. Take for three or four weeks.

MOUSEEAR

One of the outstanding remedies for whooping cough. Infuse one ounce in a pint of boiling water, and allow to stand for an hour. Strain. Dose: a tablespoonful to a wineglassful, according to age, three or four times daily. When possible administer doses following an attack of coughing, or the dose may be vomited. Mouseear is totally harmless. May be flavoured with Honey, brown sugar or Lemon.

MULLEIN

A most valuable remedy for respiratory disorders: coughs,

bronchitis, sore larynx, weak chest, etc. It is difficult to over-estimate the good effects of taking Mullein tea. The infusion of one ounce in a pint of boiling water is taken in tablespoonful to wineglassful doses, according to age, three or four times daily. May be mixed with other remedies for lung and bronchial troubles.

MUMPS

We recommend homoeopathic medicine for this trouble. In our experience there are four outstanding remedies: Jaborandi, Baryta Carb., Guaiacum and Phytolacca. The first two are probably the best in most cases. Give five pills of Jaborandi 3. and five of Baryta Carb. 6. alternately every hour. That is, Joborandi the first hour, Baryta the next hour, and so on. As symptoms lessen reduce the frequency of the doses. The other two remedies may be used in the same manner (same potencies) if the first two are not available. Jaborandi tea may also be used instead of homoeopathic remedies. Infuse half an ounce of the leaves in a pint of boiling water. Allow to stand for an hour. Dose: one to two teaspoonsful every two hours. If saliva flows very freely reduce the dose. Take less frequently as symptoms disperse.

MUSTARD

Used chiefly as a hot poultice for bronchitis, lung congestion and all acute local pains. Mix powdered Mustard with warm water to the consistency of ordinary table Mustard; spread on brown paper and apply where necessary. Remove when the skin has reddened and gently massage in some Olive oil. Mustard may be blended with Linseed for poultices.

Mustard should be used very sparingly as a condiment, as it is an irritant to the membranes of the stomach and intestines. While it has some tonic value for a sluggish stomach, its frequent use is not advised. Oil of Mustard is a very powerful irritant, and is often an ingredient in rubbing oils for rheumatism, etc.

An old custom in cases of fever was to apply poultices of Mustard, bread crumbs and Vinegar to the feet. This stimulated the circulation and helped to eliminate the toxic causes. Additionally, it was found that Mustard foot treatment gave much relief in cases of sciatica and rheumatism.

Half to one ounce of Mustard added to a hot bath is helpful in cases of insomnia, debility, poor circulation, nervous tension, colds and influenza. Mix the Mustard to a paste and then stir into the bath water. Use less for young children.

Hot Mustard Foot Baths are also excellent for all these purposes, and are especially valuable when the blood pressure is too high. Mix a tablespoonful of Mustard into a paste and add to a deep bowl of hot water. Bathe the feet for five to ten minutes.

Dry Mustard used as a massage powder is very stimulating and tonic in its effects. It is recommended in all cases of general debility where the skin is intact. Not advisable when there are pimples or skin defects. After a Mustard massage sponge down with warm water.

Mustard makes a good emetic in many cases of poisoning. For this purpose use up to one tablespoonful of domestic Mustard to half a pint of warm or tepid water.

MYRRH

Myrrh gum was employed as a medicine in biblical days, and is deservedly popular today as a remedy for sore throats, ulcers (internal and external), indigestion, debility and disordered blood. It possesses considerable tonic, antiseptic and healing properties. Ten drops of tincture of Myrrh shaken up in four ounces of distilled extract of Witch Hazel make a superior application for sprains, bruises, sores and wounds.

One teaspoonful of the tincutre in a glass of warm water should be used as a gargle for sore throats; and in cases of mouth ulcers hold this solution in the mouth for a minute or so several times daily.

Myrrh tones the stomach and every organ of the body, helps to eliminate toxic states and has a purifying action on the entire organism.

NAILS

Thin or brittle nails will be improved by Silica 12x. Take two tablets on rising and on retiring for several weeks. When the nails are thick, or tend to crumble, give five pills of

Graphites 12. morning and night. Diseased nails may call for Iris Florentina 30. or Ustilago 30. Five pills morning and night for a few weeks. If one fails try the other.

A mixture we have found very effective in all manner of nail troubles consists of equal parts of homoeopathic Calc. Fluor. 6., Silica 12., Iris Flor. 6., Graphites 6. and Ustilago 6. The dose, in liquid form, is five drops before meals twice or three times daily. Locally, tincture of Myrrh may be applied at invervals.

Diseased nails point to disordered blood and constitutional troubles; so it is important to give attention to the general health. (See also **Ingrowing Toe Nail**).

NASAL CATARRH

(See **Catarrh**). Menthol ointment in each nostril is helpful. (See **Menthol**).

NATIVE POSTURE

By adopting the native posture, instead of sitting on a seat, has of itself cured many severe cases of constipation. By taking this position the anus is distended, the intestines are squeezed and evacuation encouraged. Results may not take place at first, but will do so if persisted with. Use a pan on the floor, or squat on the usual seat, placing some material on the wood or plastic to prevent the shoes causing damage. Some have placed a small rail on the wall to help keep balance when in this position. The importance of this posture has come to the attention of some authorities, and some pans are now let into the floor of the W.C. with suitable hand rails for support. There is no doubt that this is nature's way for normal evacuation. Harrods of London supply special stands for use with the usual type of seat. They are quite satisfactory.

Aside from its importance in connection with bowel evacuation, this position has a powerful influence on the organism as a whole. It should be adopted when one feels faint or exhausted, and maintained for a few minutes. Hot towels may be applied to the anus at the same time (see **Bathing**).

NETTLE RASH

Give Nettle tea (see under **Nettles**). Or, use the remedy in homoeopathic form: Urtica Urens 3. Three or four pills every two hours until better, and then less frequently. Formica 3. is also a satisfactory remedy.

NETTLES

The stinging Nettle is a remedy for high blood pressure, arterial degeneration, nettle rash and rheumatism.

This herb is one of the chief sources of the chlorophyll sold by chemists for arterial and regenerative purposes. It must be pointed out that chlorophyll in its natural chemical association with other elements in the plant is a better medicine than the extracted substance. Its value for nettle rash is an example of the homoeopathic law of similars — 'like cures like'. Sufferers from chronic rheumatism have been cured, when other modern means have failed, by taking Nettle tea daily over a lengthy period of time. Evidence shows that it tones the arteries and reduces the blood pressure.

It is employed in the making of botanic beer, and may be cooked and served as a green vegetable in place of cabbage, etc.

Infuse one ounce of dried Nettles in a pint of boiling water. Let stand for an hour. Strain. Dose: a wineglassful before meals three times daily. When in season use the freshly gathered leaves and tops, and allow about an ounce to stand for an hour in warm (not boiling) water. Take a wineglassful three times daily. See also under **Burns**.

NEURALGIA

Make a tea from Scullcap, Valerian or Hops; or, a mixture of all three. Take a wineglass, warm, four times daily. We consider homoeopathic remedies for this trouble to be superior, especially when they are selected according to individual symptoms. For this purpose of remedy selection it is wise to consult a homoeopathic repertory or materia medica. However, for many cases Aconitum 3, five pills every hour, will usually produce satisfactory results. If not any better after four doses, try Arsenicum 3. and Gelsemium 3., taken alternately every hour. For neuralgia of the heart see **Angina Pectoris**.

Locally, bathe the painful area with hot water; dry quickly and massage in some Menthol ointment. Chamomile poultices are also useful.

NEURASTHENIA

Scullcap herb	½ ounce
Valerian root	½ ounce
Hops	½ ounce
Wild Yam	½ ounce

Simmer in two pints of water (not in an aluminium pot) for twenty minutes. Strain. Dose: a wineglassful before meals three times daily. Young people less according to age. This tea is excellent for all forms of nervous trouble. It tones the entire nervous system and relaxes the tense nerves.

If the nervous disorder is associated with sexual depletion add one single drop of tincture of Pulsatilla to each dose before taking.

Homoeopathic remedies are many, each based on the individual symptoms: Gelsemium, Valeriana, Arsen. Alb., Kali Phos., Silica, Kali Brom., China Arsen., Acid Phos., etc., etc. If interested in the homoeopathic philosophy make the remedy selection according to a repertory or materia medica.

Neurasthenics require psychological and/or spiritual aid. Also attention to diet, bathing, exercise, etc. Consult the subjects as given under the headings. Deep breathing exercises and nightly hot foot baths are almost always necessary to ensure speedy recovery.

NEURITIS

Treat as for Neuralgia. Ten tablets of Mag. Phos. 6x dissolved in a cup of hot water, taken in sips, is very effective. Repeat when necessary. Locally, apply any good counter-irritant: linament, Mustard poultice, etc.

NIGHT-BLOOMING CEREUS

The botanic name is Cactus Grandiflorus. It is used by the herbal and homoeopathic practitioners mainly for heart disorders, and is one of the best remedies for angina pectoris and valvular insufficiency. See the information given under Angina and Heart.

NIGHTMARE

A really hot foot bath before retiring will help to prevent bad dreams. A disordered digestion is a frequent cause, so feed sensibly. A cup of hot tea made from Hops taken before retiring will be of service in most cases. Excellent homoeopathic remedies are Ignatia 3. and Kali Brom. 6. Take four or five pills of Ignatia before meals, and Kali Brom. after meals, three times daily. Nux. Vom. 3., five pills three times daily, will be effective for over-worked business men subject to bad dreams. (See also under Insomnia.)

NIGHT SWEATS

These are due to debility or constitutional disorders. Red (garden) Sage tea is a useful remedy. Infuse an ounce in one pint of hot (not boiling) water and allow to stand for half an hour or more. Strain. Take a small wineglassful before meals, and another on retiring.

Homoeopathic Silica 6., five pills after meals, three times daily, will prove most helpful. This may be taken as well as the Sage tea. If no results, treat as for Debility; or, find and remedy the cause.

NIPPLES, SORE

Apply a pinch of powdered Gum Acacia (see Acacia) to the nipples and allow to stay on until feeding the baby. Will not harm the child in any way. Homoeopathically prepared Calendula ointment is also good. Apply after feeding baby, and wash off with warm water before feeding.

NOISES IN HEAD OR EARS

These noises can be most distressing. The cause may be blood pressure, disease of the middle ear, catarrh or even poisoning from taking quinine. If the sufferer has high blood pressure the cure lies in normalizing this. Homoeopathic China Sulph. 30. will cure many cases, especially if caused by taking quinine. Take five pills nightly for a while. Kali Brom. 30., taken in the same manner, will usually cure if China Sulph. fails. When the middle ear is a cause Jaborandi 30. is one of the best remedies. Ticking in one ear has often been cured by taking a daily dose of Zincum 30., or Zinc Brom. 30. Other simple remedies are Ferr. Phos. 6x, two tablets before meals, and Kali Mur. 6x, two tablets after meals.

NOSE BLEED

Pinch the nose between finger and thumb, and breathe through the mouth. A freshly-gathered leaf of the stinging nettle placed on the tongue and pressed against the palate usually has an almost immediate effect. During an attack tilt the head backwards and place a cold metal object at the back of the neck, or a cold sponge. Those subject to nose bleed should take two tablets of Ferr. Phos. 6x before meals, and five pills of Millifolium 1. after meals, three times daily.

When bleeding is severe, plug the nose with cotton wool, which may be used dry, or moistened with distilled extract of Witch Hazel.

Vigorous working of the jaws will be a help in causing nose bleed to stop. Making use of chewing gum will assist.

Some homoeopaths recommend Chelidonium 30, five pills every ten minutes until six doses have been taken, but cease if the bleeding stops before the six doses have been taken. As a preventative take a dose once daily for a few days. Chelidonium should be most effective where the sufferer is subject to liver upset.

NUTMEG

A splendid remedy for a weak digestion with flatulence. Effective in material doses, or in homoeopathic potency. A good pinch of powdered Nutmeg in a little hot, sweetened water after meals will usually end a bout of flatulence. For chronic flatulence take five pills of Nux Mosc. 3. (Nutmeg) before every meal for some weeks.

NUX VOMICA

This is a poison, but when prepared homoeopathically it loses all poisonous effects from the 3rd. potency upwards. Even a low potency of 2x can do no harm. Nux Vom. covers a very wide field of action. It is a remarkable remedy when it meets the symptoms, and will produce outstanding results in cases of indigestion, debility, nervous exhaustion, impotency and when one is 'out-of-sorts'. Any tired person can safely give Nux Vom. a trial for a week or so. Take five pills of the 3rd. potency before meals, three times daily.

OAK

Medicine prepared from Oak bark or acorns is strongly antiseptic and astringent; hence, it is useful for sore throats, septic conditions and diarrhoea. It also possesses some tonic value, and some practitioners use it in powder form as an ingredient in herbal Composition Powder. The tincture is suggested as the most pleasant form in which this valuable medicine can be taken: half a teaspoonful in warm water, well sweetened with Honey, before meals. A smaller dose of five to ten drops in hot water before meals is good for disorders of the spleen, and this is especially suitable for those who suffer from an excess of alcohol.

As a gargle for sore throat use a teaspoonful of the tincture in a tumbler of tepid water. For diarrhoea take half a teaspoonful in tepid water every three hours until better. A teaspoonful to a pint of warm water makes an excellent injection for leucorrhoea.

OATS

There are several varieties of Oats, and all are excellent food for brain and nerves. The best is the Black Oat. The medicinal tincture known as Avena Sativa is made from this latter variety. The stimulating effect of Oats on horses is well known, and it should have similar effects on human beings. The old herbalists produced some wonderful cures in cases of nervous debility, nervous dyspepsia and lassitude with this remedy, and such cures are still taking place. Symptoms due to loss of nerve power will often respond to this simple food-remedy.

Unfortunately, Oat tincture is not always made properly. The chief medicinal value lies in the Oat 'whiskers' and resinous gum found on the outer covering of the Black Oat. Some tinctures are made from the grain only; and, while this has its value, the main medicinal virtues are not present. Twenty to thirty drops of good Oat tincture will give more energy than a glass of brandy, without any of the alcoholic effects. It is indeed a superior nerve tonic and food. An ideal preparation may be made at home. Place one pint of Black Oats with three pints of distilled water (or, water that has been boiled and allowed to cool) in an earthenware jar. Add two ounces of glycerine. Cover the jar, and simmer gently down to about one quart. Strain the liquid through muslin, or a fine sieve, and bottle ready for use. This medicine will be quite good if made from whole Black Oats only; but, if it is possible, add the Oat 'whiskers' as well, when it will be even more effective.

Take a wineglass of this infusion, hot, three times daily; or, whenever a stimulant is called for. Take for nerviness, fatigue, loss of nerve power over the muscles, at the first symptoms of a cold or when mentally depressed. Ideal for weakly children and invalids. The flavour may be improved by adding fruit juice, or a good pinch of Cinnamon.

OBESITY

In most cases careful attention to diet will do much to reduce weight; in others it appears not to make any difference at all. Some women have gone on starvation diets to lose weight, and have almost destroyed themselves in the process. The fact has to be faced that putting on flesh is natural for some types, just as others will always be thin, no matter how or what they eat. There is plenty of evidence to show that thin folk have a greater expectancy of long life than have the fat. Fat people are more subject to heart and circulatory trouble, thrombosis, etc. Many cases of obesity can be traced to a faulty thyroid gland, and this is probably why that great constituional remedy, Kelp, will often do much to reduce weight, as it contains iodine and has a direct action on the thyroid. As thinness can sometimes be traced to imbalance of the thyroid, it follows that the thin may take this food-remedy without doing any harm. Kelp may be tried in crude or homoeopathic form, as good results follow no matter how it is taken. However, for deeply-seated constitutional trouble and obesity it is suggested in the 30th. potency: five pills morning and night.

Phytolacca 30. (five pills twice daily) may succeed in those cases where Kelp (Fucus) fails to produce results. In any case fat people with arterial trouble, heart disorders and a tendency to blood clotting should take a dose of Cholesterin 30. for some weeks, a few minutes before the midday meal.

In these days all stout people know that they should cut down starchy food. Sugar should be eliminated from the diet, and pure Honey taken instead, even for sweetening beverages.

Bread should be replaced by rye biscuits such as 'Ryvita'. If possible eliminate cake, pastry, fried food, cooked animal and processed fats. Be easy on potatoes, and have them baked or boiled in their jackets. The best cooking oils are from maize or sunflower seed; or Linseed oil is good.

Keep the bowels regular (see **Constipation**).

Don't worry about putting on weight. Worry will make the thin lose more flesh, and cause the stout to put it on. Strenuous exercise is not likely to be of much help in most cases, but a reasonable amount of activity, especially sharp walking, is good for all.

OINTMENTS

A great deal of rubbish has been written about ointments as a cure for wounds, sores and skin diseases. Some, containing suppressive chemicals, do a great deal of harm, driving poisons that are trying to come out of the system via the skin back into the organism. Suppressive treatment of skin trouble often results in the development of serious internal disorders. The skin trouble is not cured, but suppressed. All real cure must come by and through the blood.

Ointments that do not suppress, and which consist of harmless ingredients, have their uses. The use of Menthol ointment has been described elsewhere. Herbal ointments prepared from Marigold, Marshmallow, Comfrey, St. John's Wort and other herbs have done good work for sores, wounds, ulcers and skin diseases. There is no doubt that these ointments enable the system to take up some of the healing virtues they possess. Even if a natural ointment does not do anything more than keep the area clean it will serve a good purpose. Marigold (Calendula) ointment is one of the best for general purposes, and it can be made at home. Gather fresh Marigold petals. Melt half a pound of white petroleum jelly, or lanolin in a large earthenware jar. An iron or stainless steel saucepan will do if a suitable jar is not available. Stir in as large a quantity of the Marigold petals as the melted fat will take, and allow to stew for half an hour. Strain off, place in any jar of sufficient size, and add immediately about a teaspoonful of oil of Eucalyptus. Stir every few minutes until the preparation begins to cool. This ointment is good for

sores, wounds, ulcers, varicose veins, skin disorders, bruises,
etc. Owing to the presence of the Eucalyptus do not get it
into the eyes, although no harm will be done if this happens
when applying to sore lids.

OLIVE OIL

An excellent dressing for salads. Add Lemon juice as well
instead of Vinegar. Olive oil is nutritious. It helps the liver in
many cases and is a very gentle laxative. For the latter reason
it is excellent for children. The oil is very soothing to the
membranes of the stomach and bowels, and appears to exert
a pleasing influence on the nervous system. Olive oil is also
very good when employed for massage. Massage of the thin
and nervy with Olive oil is an aid to nutrition.

Many cannot take the oil internally, but they can do so if
it is emulsified. Mr. W. G. Orr discovered the virtues of
emulsified Olive oil during the first world war, when it
proved a most valuable restorative food for shell-shocked
soldiers. We, personally, have known it to prove wonderfully
helpful for neurasthenics and sufferers from malnutrition. By
emulsifying the oil its particles are split up and the oil
absorbed and utilized by the system without upsetting the
liver. Mr. Orr originally used malted milk powder. One or two
teaspoonsful of best Olive oil were mixed with a tablespoonful or more of the powdered milk, and hot milk, or part milk
and water, added. This was then well shaken in a jar. Now,
with high speed kitchen mixers available, the shaking up in a
jar is unnecessary. Emulsified oil will prevent, and occasionally cure, gall stones.

A tumblerful of this emulsified oil and milk is a meal in
itself. The sick and debilitated should try it, two or three
times daily. It is delicious. Take slowly for the best effects.

ONION

Cooked Onions are an old cure for coughs and colds, and a
most effective one for those who can take Onions without
them disagreeing. Onion syrup is also good for coughs,
asthma and bronchitis. The Onion is antiseptic and purifies
the blood. Probably the best way to use the Onion (Allium
Cepa) medicinally for colds is to take it in the 3rd.
homoeopathic potency: four or five pills every two hours at

the onset of a cold; but note that only that type of cold associated with running nose and watering of the eyes will positively respond to this medicine. Here we have an example of the homoeopathic law at work. Smell an Onion, and the eyes water, the nose runs and one feels distressed -- the symptoms of a type of cold in the head. As the raw Onion produces exactly those symptoms, it will cure a cold with those symptoms when taken in minute doses. It has been said that to merely sniff a cut Onion will sometimes cure a cold in the very early stages. Also, that a cut Onion in a saucer, placed in a room, will prevent and cure colds.

OPERATIONS

The science of surgery is so advanced that much of the risk and fear formerly associated with operations have been removed. The skill of the modern surgeon is amazing; although we have to confess that many operations could be avoided. Surgery is an admission that medicine has failed. During long experience we have found that a short course of homoeopathic Kali Phos. 30. before an operation will do a great deal to prepare the sufferer in mind and body for the event, and promote healing afterwards. Kali Phos. gives strength to brain, nerves and tissues, and it is also a remedy for fear states. Take five pills of Kali Phos. 30. morning and night for a week before the operation. Doses may be resumed for a short period after surgery has been performed, when circumstances permit. Another wonderful remedy for the after-effects of operations on the abdominal organs is Vanadium 30. Both Kali Phos. and Vanadium deal with shock. So, if an operation has been performed on the abdomen we advise five pills of Kali Phos. 30. in the morning, and five of Vanadium 30. in the evening as soon after the event as is possible, and to be continued for two or three weeks.

ORANGE

Similar to the Lemon (see **Lemon**), but not so powerful. A few people cannot tolerate oranges, and they should not be taken by such.

ORRIS

The powdered root is used, on account of its fragrancy, in toilet and dental powders. Homoeopathically prepared it becomes a powerful medicine for many ailments, including nerve troubles affecting the nerve endings, diseases of the nasal membranes, weakness of the aorta, vein troubles, duodenal disorders and diseased nails.

Take four or five pills of the 30th. potency morning and night for any of the troubles mentioned. We have found it especially valuable in cases of duodenal ulcer, although it is not the best remedy in all cases.

OSTEOPATHY

This splendid manipulative science is coming more and more into its own. So many ailments are due wholly, or in part, to defects and subluxations in the bony structure, especially in the spine. Unfortunately there are many so-called osteopaths who have had no proper training, and there is no doubt that some of these gentry have done harm to their patients and to the science itself. Not all qualified osteopaths are good osteopaths; even as not all doctors are good doctors. Likewise, some manipulative practitioners who do not hold a D.O. degree are better than some who do. However, unless a practitioner has a very good name, it is wise to seek the services of a fully qualified man who is a member of one of the recognized schools, or is on the Register of Osteopaths. Look for D.O. and M.R.O., or, see if the one who has D.O. only after his name has been trained at a reputable college.

Osteopaths say that structure governs function, and this is undoubtedly true. It is also true to say that function determines structure — nature teaches us that! Hence, not all cases respond to osteopathy, even as not all respond to wise medication. So often a corrected spinal bone will slip back into its faulty position very soon after treatment, because the basic cause in nerves and muscles has not been eliminated. We have known scores of cases of spinal subluxation cured by means of carefully selected remedies; and, we have also had cases which would not respond without manipulation.

In skilled hands, osteopathy can only do good; and all people would be better for such attention at intervals during their lives, for 'a stitch in time saves nine'.

PAIN

'Oh doctor, at times I have such a pain in my side! I'm sure I've got heart trouble'. Diagnosis revealed, not heart disease, but a serious splenic condition which called for immediate attention. But for the pain the patient would never have known that anything was wrong, and she would have died suddenly, at a later date. Pain was nature's warning that something was wrong. We only experience pain when an abnormal or subnormal condition exists, so it is useless treating the pain itself; attention must be given to the cause. It will thus be seen that even to treat a headache with suppressive drugs cannot remove the reason why the headache was present in the first place. Also, the drug will only add to the underlying causes. Of course there are circumstances when drugs may be essential, although they are not nearly so frequent as may be thought. There are many natural ways of conquering pain, but in all instances the cause must be treated as well as the discomfort itself. Of course, to remove the cause will take away the effects, although it may take some time to accomplish the former in certain cases, when both the disorder and the resultant pain must receive attention. Counter-irritants are among the best pain remedies, even as they were four thousand years ago.

Hot fomentations, packs, poultices and ointments may be employed to relieve pain in circumstances calling for such external attention. Harmless pain-killing herbs are Scullcap, Chamomile, Valerian, Hops and nerve herbs generally. A great number of homoeopathic remedies deal effectively with pain, among them being Aconitum, Gelsemium, Chamomilla, Belladonna, Ferr. Phos. and Mag. Phos.

Pain may be relieved by suggestive therapy or hypnotism, but these practices can, in some instances, be as harmful as suppression by drugs unless the cause also receives attention.

Pain, like all suffering, has psychological values. The fierce discipline of pain often gives birth to wisdom.

PALPITATION

May be due to heart weakness, debility or digestive trouble. Treat the cause (see the headings).

PARSLEY

Parsley is well-known as an article of use for culinary purposes. Its wonderful medicinal properties are not so well appreciated. It is carminative, diuretic and resolvent. That is to say it helps the stomach, tones the urinary organs and gives great relief in glandular swellings and tissue derangements when used locally as a poultice. Made into a tea it will help to dissolve stone in the kidneys and bladder, relieve flatulence and comfort the abdominal organs. It will also do much to normalize female irregularities; but should not be taken, except in small quantities, by pregnant women.

Applied locally, it will cleanse open wounds and has few equals for treating sore places caused by injuries from rusty nails and metals. Also good for bruises and inflamed joints. Bruised Parsley laid on the eyes is very soothing and healing when they are inflamed. Use also for the bites and stings of insects.

The tea is made by placing a good handful of fresh Parsley in a jug and pouring on a pint of hot (not boiling) water. After thirty minutes or so it is ready to be taken in wineglassful doses before meals. The dried herb may be so used when the fresh is not available.

For sores, stings and wounds apply as a cold poultice, after rubbing up with the leaves. For glandular swellings rub up enough to make a poultice to cover the affected area. Renew every four hours. One such poultice may be kept on all night.

PARSLEY PIERT

Similar in action to garden Parsley, but stronger. This is one of the best remedies possible for stone, gravel, kidney and bladder complaints. It used to be prescribed very frequently by medical men before modern drugs clouded their knowledge of nature's own remedies. Doses for internal use the same as for garden Parsley. If the dried herb is employed allow the infusion to stand for an hour before using.

PASSION FLOWER

A fine remedy for nervous irritability, insomnia, neuralgia, hysteria, nervous headaches, bronchial asthma and spasmodic conditions. The dose is ten to twenty drops of the fluid extract in some hot water, three times daily. We have found better and quicker results follow the taking of the fresh plant tincture (from homoeopathic chemists), when the dose need be only five or six drops in a teaspoonful of cold or tepid water. For insomnia take before meals and again on retiring. The most satisfactory results can be anticipated from taking this remedy, but it should be continued for some time.

PEACE

When the mind is at peace, the body is tranquil. Pain and irritation in the physical organism causes mental restlessness.

The mind and body work in unison and mental processes often affect the physical, causing a wide variety of ailments. 'As a man thinketh, so he is'.

The harbouring of destructive thoughts and emotions associated with anger, resentment, jealousy, etc., causes many illnesses.

By banishing from the mind thoughts that are opposed to peace is an enormous stride towards health and happiness. (Read what is said under **Psychology** and **Spiritual Aid**).

PEACH

Both the bark and the leaves are used in medicine. It is a fine remedy for irritation and congestion of the gastric surfaces, and has been found to be of great benefit in nervous dyspepsia, inflamed stomach and intestines, vomiting and "irritable conditions'. There are few better remedies for the morning sickness of pregnancy. Peach tea is also good for bronchitis and coughs; especially for whooping cough. Infuse half an ounce of the bark, or one ounce of the leaves, in a pint of boiling water. Allow to stand for half an hour. Dose: a teaspoonful to a tablespoonful, according to age and requirements, three times daily.

PELLITORY-OF-THE-WALL

One of the proven remedies for kidney and bladder disorders. There are many herbs for all the various ailments, and all are good. The sufferer may, therefore, use whatever remedy is obtainable with confidence. The infusion of the herb is one ounce to a pint of boiling water. Take a small wineglassful before or after meals, three times daily, for kidney and bladder weakness, stone, gravel and suppression of the urine.

PENNYROYAL

This remedy has been employed chiefly as a female medicine for obstructed menstruation; and for this it is excellent, especially when the trouble is due to a chill. It is also good for spasms, hysteria, stomach weakness and flatulence. Most valuable for the colds of children. Infuse an ounce in a pint of boiling water and allow to stand for at least fifteen minutes before taking. Do not boil or simmer this herb. The adult dose is a small teacupful, taken warm, every two or three hours; rather more frequently for colds and chills. Give children less according to age, and sweeten with honey if desired.

There are, however, other uses for this remedy when it is taken in homoeopathic potency. Five pills of Mentha Pulegium in the 30th. potency, taken night and morning, are excellent for simple anaemia, splenic trouble, ovarian pains, piles when the veins are much affected, duodenal weakness and ulcers. The writer's long experience proves beyond all doubt the great value of Pennyroyal in these cases. We cannot speak too highly of this remedy.

PEONY

An antispasmodic and tonic; useful in chorea, nervous disorders and spasmodic affections. The infusion of one ounce of powdered root in one pint of boiling water is taken in wineglassful doses. Minute doses of the fresh plant tincture, or of the 3rd. homoeopathic potency, will often cure haemorrhoids and fissures in the rectum; especially when there is itching, burning and swelling. This is a remedy which can be resorted to when other medicines for piles and rectal troubles fail to produce the necessary results. Take three or four drops of the fresh plant tincture, or five pills of Paeonia 3., before meals, three times daily.

PEPPERMINT

One of the most useful and effective remedies for indigestion of a simple character; flatulence, sickness and general digestive upsets. When combined with Elder Flowers it is excellent for colds and fevers (see **Elder Flowers**). As a beverage, Peppermint tea, made in a pot, is vastly superior to ordinary tea as a healthful and refreshing drink. Sweeten to taste and add Lemon if desired. Menthol is obtained from Peppermint oil. A few drops of essence of Peppermint in warm sweetened water, is usually all that is necessary to bring comfort and relief in the stomach upsets of children; and, very often, to adults as well.

PERITONITIS

The services of a professional healer are most strongly advised. Until such services are at hand give five pills of Aconitum 3. every hour. Bryonia and Gelsemium are also helpful remedies. Flannels soaked in equal parts of hot water and Vinegar should be applied to the abdomen frequently.

PERIWINKLE

The Greater Periwinkle has been found to be a good remedy for anaemia, female period pains and pancreatic weakness. Infuse an ounce of the herb in a pint of boiling water. Allow to stand for half an hour. Dose: a wineglassful before meals. Children less according to age.

PERUVIAN BARK

For a very long time Peruvian bark was considered to be the best remedy for malaria and fevers with similar symptoms. Quinine is prepared from this remedy, and although the preparation has a powerful action, it can do much harm and is not nearly so valuable as the natural, untreated medicine. We are always contacting cases of quinine poisoning. Hahnemann, the founder of homoeopathy, noticed that quinine produced the very symptoms it was supposed to cure; so he came to the conclusion that minute doses instead of the usual large quantities prescribed, would achieve far better results, not only in the treatment of malaria but in all cases where symptoms due to, or similar to, quinine poisoning were manifested. How right he was! Homoeopathic doses of this valuable remedy are excellent for malaria, fevers of the malarial character, general debility, disorders resulting from sexual abuse, indigestion, neuralgia, headaches, giddiness and ringing in the ears.

The infusion, or the ordinary tincture, will also produce the most pleasing results; but the dose should be small. Place an ounce of the cut bark in a jug, add a pint of boiling water and allow to stand for two hours. Give one to two teaspoonsful of the medicine every hour for intermittent fevers, colds and acute conditions. Or, for indigestion and as a constitutional tonic, a similar dose before every meal. The dose of the tincture is five to ten drops in water; frequency according to the conditions, as for the infusion. When there is flatulence, and Peruvian bark is taken as a medicine, a little Cinnamon should be added to each dose; this also applies to the treatment of influenza.

Experience has taught us that this remedy, which is commonly called China, has a better action when taken in homoeopathic potency. For fevers take five pills of the 3rd potency every hour until better. As a tonic and digestive take before meals. In cases of great debility and exhaustion use the 30th potency: five pills on rising and again on retiring.

PILES

Piles (haemorrhoids) are a very distressing affliction, causing pain, annoyance and loss of vitality. Generally speaking, the condition points to a history of constipation and the taking of purgatives; although a few cases have come to our attention where there has never been any costive condition. In any case the diet must receive attention and the bowels kept open with a laxative breakfast (See **Diet**).

Some suppositories are good, and others are harmful. It is wise to obtain suppositories from a health or herbal store, in which case the ingredients are effective but harmless. Suppositories containing Witch Hazel or Pilewort are always reliable, and may be used at the same time as constitutional treatment is given. An old remedy was to use a peeled clove of Garlic as a suppository. Insert it at night. If the clove goes right in it will be evacuated with the first motion.

Here is an old cure which acts in most cases: Shred up one or two ounces of freshly gathered Pilewort roots. Add to half a pint of new milk, and bring to the boil. Eat the whole on retiring. In some cases one such dose is sufficient to cure; in others it may have to be repeated two or three times. The fluid extract of Pilewort is also quite good, but not nearly so effective as the fresh roots. If using the extract take a teaspoonful in hot milk or water on retiring and before breakfast for several days. The extract may also be applied with the finger three or four times daily. Green Pilewort Ointment, sold by herbal vendors, is ideal. Apply two or three times daily.

The fluid extract of Stone Root is also effective. Take 20 to 30 drops with Honey in a little warm water after meals. While on this remedy keep the bowels open if necessary with a mild laxative. Another recommended remedy is fluid extract of Canadian Pine: apply a little with the finger three times daily, and take ten drops in a little water before or after meals.

Reliable homoeopathic remedies are Aesculus Hip. 3, Collinsonia 3, and Hamamelis 3. Either may be tried. Dose: five pills before meals three times daily.

Honey, used as an ointment, may be applied and inserted into the back passage two or three times daily. Good results have been claimed for this.

PILEWORT

The Pilewort (Lesser Celandine) is a great remedy for piles (See under Piles).

PINE

There are several types of Pine, and the one usually referred to is Pinus Sylvestris from which turpentine is obtained. The oil is used medicinally for chronic affections of the kidneys and bladder. Two or three drops with brown sugar or Honey may be taken three times daily at meal times. Much good has been accomplished with this simple remedy in urinary disorders; also for chronic bronchial affections. If results are not obtained within a few days we do not advise the sufferer to continue with the remedy. Oil of Pine is also a very good external treatment for wounds which will not heal, abscesses etc. As a liniment it is excellent for painful muscles and joints. Also good for Lumbago, when two-drop doses should also be taken internally in brown sugar or Honey. The famous 'Dutch Drops' for kidney and bladder trouble and back pains, are prepared as follows: Spirits of Turpentine, one gill; Oil of Juniper, half an ounce; Flowers of Sulphur, one ounce. Shake well and keep in a warm place for a week. Dose: ten to fifteen drops in brown sugar or Honey three times daily.

PINK ROOT
Simmer one ounce in a pint of water for 15 minutes. Strain. This is a reliable worm medicine. The dose for children is a tablespoonful morning and night. Adults, a large wineglassful. A herbal laxative should also be taken with the nightly dose.

Pink Root in homoeopathic form is a recognised remedy for Angina Pectoris. Take four or five pills of Pink Root (Spigelia) 30. morning and night.

PINUS BARK (Canadian Pine)
This is a powerful tonic and astringent medicine, and is usually one of the ingredients in Composition Powder. A pile remedy.

PLANTAIN
The fresh leaves, rubbed on insect stings and bites, afford instant relief. Bruised leaves, held in the mouth, will sometimes relieve toothache. Homoeopathic Plantago 3. in liquid form is ideal for toothache, earache and neuralgia. Take five drops in a dry spoon every hour until better, and then less frequently. A few drops of the mother tincture of the fresh plant (Plantago ϕ) on a handkerchief, applied to the painful area, will often afford great relief in neuralgia. Some writers consider Plantago ϕ to be a good remedy for neurasthenia: three or four drops in tepid water, three times daily.

PLEURISY
The following medicine is recommended:

Pleurisy root	½ ounce
Scullcap herb	½ ounce
Ginger in powder	¼ teaspoonful.

Simmer gently in a pint of water for 15 minutes, using an iron or enamel pot. Strain. Take a tablespoonful to a wineglassful, according to age, every three hours, and less frequently as the condition improves. May be flavoured with Lemon and/or Honey. Chamomile fomentations, or Linseed or Bran poultices may be applied to the chest. Follow with hot Olive oil rubs.

The homoeopathic treatment consists of four or five pills of Aconitum 3x. and Bryonia 3x. taken alternately every two hours. As the temperature drops gradually reduce the frequency of the Aconitum and finally discontinue it; but keep on with the Bryonia until well. There are several other suitable remedies for the treatment of pleurisy, but those given will meet the requirements of most cases. In all cases where fever is present keep the sufferer off solid food, and administer plenty of fresh Lemon juice.

PLEURISY ROOT

A most valuable remedy for pleurisy, bronchitis and coughs. It promotes expectoration, relieves difficult breath-ing and is very soothing to the lungs and nervous system. It has a mild tonic action, and adds to the sufferer's vitality. Simmer half an ounce of the crushed root in a pint of water for 15 minutes. Strain. The average dose is a wineglassful every two or three hours, taken warm and sweetened. Or, take as given under Pleurisy.

PNEUMONIA

The herbal formula given under Pleurisy has been found very effective. A satisfactory homoeopathic method is to give four or five pills of Aconitum 3x. every hour for ten hours; then four or five pills of Phosphorus 6. every two hours in alternation with Aconitum 3x. That is to say, a dose of Aconitum at 8 a.m., Phosphorus at 10 a.m., Aconitum at 12 noon, Phosphorus at 2 p.m., and so on, for one day. The day following give five pills of Bryonia 3. and five of Antimonium Tart. 6. alternately every two hours, and continue the two latter remedies until the trouble has cleared. (See also under Bryonia).

Hot Linseed poultices should be applied to the chest and back, and renewed when cool. Give plenty of hot Lemon and Honey. Wise people will seek the services of a skilled healer for accurate diagnosis and treatment; but the remedies advised can only do good, and should produce the most satisfactory results.

POISON OAK
See under **Rhus Tox**.

POISONING
Administer an emetic of one or two teaspoonsful of powdered Mustard in a pint of tepid water — the patient to swallow as much as he can. If necessary, tickle the back of the tongue to induce vomiting. Another good emetic is a teaspoonful of Ipecacuanha Wine in a little water every ten minutes until vomiting is induced. If carbolic acid is the poison taken, give plenty of Olive oil. **Send for the doctor.**

POKE ROOT
Employed as a herbal remedy for dyspepsia, rheumatism, dysmenorrhoea, scabies, ringworm and blood disorders. The dose is half a teaspoonful of the fluid extract in hot water three times daily. Taken in homoeopathic form it is one of the most valuable remedies it is possible to take for inflammation and lumps in the female breasts. Taken alternately with Hemlock (Conium Mac.) it is doubtful whether any better system of medication is possible. See under **Hemlock**. For this purpose use the 30th potency. Poke root (Phytolacca) in the 3rd potency is also excellent for sore throats. Take four pills every hour until easier, and then less frequently.

POLYPUS (Nasal)
Take five pills of Thuja 30. morning and night, and two tablets of Kali Mur. 6x. after meals, three times daily. Paint the polypus once daily with Thuja ϕ. (The symbol ϕ means the strong mother tincture as supplied by homoeopathic chemists).

If the above treatment fails try five pills of Agraphis Nutans 3. before meals, and five of Sticta 3. after meals, three times daily. In all cases take Kali Mur. 6x after meals. It goes well with the Sticta.

Yet another treatment should either of the above fail: Five

pills of Teucrium 3. before meals; two tablets of Kali Mur. 6x after meals, three times daily. Paint the polypus with Teucrium φ once daily; or, get powdered Teucrium and use it as a snuff, two or three times daily. Bad cases should seek professional advice. The treatment advised for **Adenoids** has also proved effective.

POMEGRANATE

One of the oldest known remedies for tapeworm. Eight ounces of the coarse root-bark boiled in three pints of water for half an hour. Strain, and then boil the liquid for another hour, or down to about one pint. Add a little Molasses. Give the patient a small teacupful followed by a dose of Epsom salts, or any purgative. Repeat four hours later if necessary.

Taken as a homoeopathic remedy it is useless for worms, but one of the finest remedies for auto-toxaemia ever discovered. For those who believe in the germ theory we can say that it destroys bacterium coli, and removes the reasons why the bacteria are present! The best results have followed taking high potencies. In all cases of bowel toxaemia the following is advised: take five pills of Pomegranate (Granatum) 200. on rising, again on retiring and a final dose on rising the next morning. The day after take a dose of Granatum 30. on rising and again on retiring, and continue taking two doses daily for three weeks. When toxaemia is at the back of any kind of illness and debility, this medicine may produce astonishing results. It is totally harmless and well worth trying.

POPLAR (White)

Many experienced herbalists regard the Poplar as being superior to Peruvian Bark (Cinchona) as a general tonic to the entire system. Unlike the latter, a medicine made from Poplar bark is unlikely to produce undesirable effects, even when taken for some lengthy period in material doses.

The fluid extract is a convenient form in which to take this excellent remedy. It is deservedly popular for indigestion, especially when the stomach lacks tone. Also for flatulence, acidity, nausea, difficult urination, scalding urine, enlarged prostate gland, catarrh of the bladder, ague and night sweats. The dose is half to one teaspoonful in hot water before or after meals. Here is a very good digestive and constitutional tonic:

Fluid extract Poplar	1 ounce
Fluid extract Wild Yam	½ ounce
Tincture Cardomoms Co	2 ounces

Dose: one to two teaspoonsful in warm water before meals, or as required. Children less according to age.

POPPY (Red)

Heat one pound of Honey and stir in as many freshly gathered Poppy petals as the Honey will take. Simmer for ten minutes, giving an occasional stir. Strain into a jar whilst warm. This forms a very fine medicine for coughs and nervous irritability. Give a teaspoonful whenever a cough is troublesome. Quite often a teaspoonful on retiring promotes sleep. Adults may take up to two teaspoonful doses. Opium, which is obtained from the Eastern Poppy is positively not advisable for home use, and can only be obtained when prescribed by a medical man. However, Opium in homoeopathic form is one of the best liver tonics. Three or four pills of Opium 3 are taken before meals for sluggish liver and resultant constipation. In this form Opium is totally harmless. We often prescribe it in the 3rd or 30th potency for liver troubles when a medicine such as Mandrake (Podophyllum) fails; and with most satisfactory results.

POSTURE

The human engine can only function at its best when the body is held in the correct posture. This applies to standing, walking and sitting. Keep the crown of the head high, the chin in, chest out and abdomen in. Do not practice this in a tensed, military fashion, but in a positive, relaxed manner. Read what is said on this subject under **Breathing and Exercise.**

POTATO

Those who are better for not taking too much starchy food can usually deal with the Potato better than with bread. We would remind those who run down the humble spud that in poor country districts, especially in Ireland, people live almost exclusively on them, and manage to keep as fit as the average person. A quantity of valuable mineral salts are found in Potato peel, and to obtain the full value of the mineral content Potatoes should be either baked or boiled in their jackets.

Raw Potato juice is good for rheumatism. One or two teaspoonsful of the juice pressed out of mashed raw Potato, and taken before meals, will do much to eliminate an acid condition and remove a reason for rheumatic ailments.

In some country areas it has been, and still is, the custom for rheumatic sufferers to carry a Potato in their pocket. It is claimed that the Potato will take unto itself some of the rheumatism (acid) from which the person suffers. A farm labourer who had been a great rheumatic sufferer told the writer that carrying a Potato about had cured him completely, and that he always carried one with him to keep the trouble away. Maybe there were other reasons for the cure; but there is sufficient evidence of there being something in the idea for us to suggest it to sufferers. After a few days the old Potato should be thrown away and replaced by a new one.

Potato pulp forms a wonderful dressing for sores and septic wounds. We recall curing a badly wounded and septic thumb with a cold raw Potato poultice in the case of a working man whose doctor had advised amputation of the member. One merely applies cold pulped or scraped Potato to the sore or wound, and bandages it in position; never too tightly. Renew every six to eight hours.

Another way to treat rheumatism and blood disorders is to thoroughly wash Potato peelings and boil them for a few minutes. Strain, and take a wineglassful three or four times daily. This has been known to cure rheumatism, fibrositis, skin diseases, and blood disorders in general. In the old days, when sailing ships crossed the oceans, and the sailors were without fresh vegetables and fruits for weeks and months at a time, outbreaks of scurvy and disorders due to mineral salt deficiency were common, often reaching alarming heights. The old captains had one never-failing cure for the men — the water in which Potato peelings had been boiled.

Scraped Potato is excellent for burns.

POULTICES

Here are some very fine poultices for coughs, bronchitis, neuralgia, congestions and pains in general.

Bran

Prepare a flannel or linen bag of the size required to well cover the area to be treated. Fill it loosely with Bran. Pour boiling water over this until thoroughly moistened. Place in a towel and wring fairly dry. Apply as soon as it has cooled enough for the patient to bear without discomfort. Apply to the base of the spine for sciatica.

Bread

Place half a pint of boiling water into a large basin, and add as much crumbled Bread as the water will take. Place a plate over the basin and keep covered for about ten minutes. Pour off the water, but do not squeeze the Bread mass. Spread evenly on linen and apply to the part. This is quite good for pains and swellings, splinters in the fingers, etc.

Chamomile

Scald Chamomile flowers (or the herb) with boiling water and apply on linen. Excellent for faceache, neuralgia, neuritis, etc. More convenient if used in a bag as suggested for Bran.

Charcoal

Prepare bread as for a bread poultice, but stir in gently one or two ounces of powdered wood Charcoal. This is very good for foul wounds and offensive ulcers.

Chest Poultice

Chop up six fair-sized Onions. Add about the same quantity of rye meal or oatmeal. Mix with sufficient Vinegar to form a thick paste. Heat over the fire for five to ten minutes. Place the mixture in a linen bag large enough to cover the chest, and apply as hot as possible. Before the poultice gets cold apply another. Repeat again if necessary. Bran, Linseed or Mustard may also be employed for pneumonia with good effect.

Finely cut raw onion applied as a cold poultice to the upper part of the chest and kept on all night is excellent for colds, coughs and bronchitis.

Linseed

Place a small quantity of Linseed meal into a warm basin. Add a little boiling water, and stir briskly so that the mixture is free from lumps. Spread thickly on linen and apply to the area as hot as the patient can bear. Renew if necessary when cold.

Mustard

Mix Mustard with hot water to the consistency of table Mustard. Spread on linen or brown paper, and apply as desired. See also **Mustard**. Never leave a Mustard plaster or poultice on for more than 20 minutes.

Slippery Elm Poultice

Powdered Slippery Elm	2 parts.
Lobelia seed	1 part.
Ground Ginger	1 part.

Mix thoroughly with hot water, and apply direct to the part. Cover with towelling.

This poultice is good for anything from stiff and swollen joints to chest complaints. If there is much hardness or swelling add to the mixture one or two teaspoonsful of chloride of potassium. Plain Slippery Elm also makes a most satisfactory poultice.

NOTE: If the skin be smeared with glycerine before applying a poultice this will prevent the particles from adhering to the flesh.

A HEALING PLASTER

Spread a thin layer of petroleum jelly, as one would apply butter to bread, over a piece of brown paper or white linen of sufficient size to cover the area to be treated, but leave a margin of about half an inch clear of the jelly. Well sprinkle with powdered Comfrey Root, a pepper pot may be used for this purpose. Apply over wounds, inflamed areas and ulcers, and renew every twenty four hours, or sooner. For the treatment of painful areas where the skin is not broken the

powdered Comfrey may be blended with an equal part of
Cayenne pepper. Most helpful for painful muscles and joints.
When Cayenne is used the plaster may have to be taken off
after a shorter period if there is discomfort. Skin sensitively
differs considerably and some can tolerate applications of
counter-irritants much longer than others.

PREGNANCY

Cut or rub up finely equal parts of dried Raspberry leaves
and Motherwort herb. Use this instead of ordinary tea, but a
rather larger quantity. Prepare in a teapot (not aluminium).
The tea should be taken at least three times daily. Sweeten,
or add Lemon as desired. This helpful beverage should be
taken for at least three months before delivery. It helps in
every possible manner, strengthening and normalising the
organs and giving strength to the prospective mother. When
making allow to stand for at least 15 minutes before pouring.
One to three teacupsful may be taken at a time.

In cases of habitual or threatened abortion, five pills of
homoeopathic Actaea Racemosa 3. should be taken before
meals, and five of Aletris Far. 3. after meals, three times daily
for the first two months, and for the last two months. See
also **Morning Sickness.**

A great deal of harm is done by sexual intercourse during
pregnancy, both the mother and the unborn suffer, and quite
often birth is made difficult. Restraint and great moderation is
called for, and the husband should have enough sense to be
guided by the wife's feelings in the matter. Animals avoid
intercourse during pregnancy.

Those who prefer biochemic remedies should take two
tablets of Calc. Phos. 3x before meals, two of Calc. Fluor. 6x
after meals, and two of Kali. Phos. 6x on rising and on
retiring. These biochemic tissue salts will give strength to the
prospective mother and supply her and the growing babe with
the vital calcium and potassium necessary to health and the
growth of strong bone. There is no need to take both
homoeopathic and biochemic remedies; but the herbal tea may
be taken as well if desired.

PRICKLY ASH

Both the bark and the berries of this tree are used in

medicine. It is one of the finest general tonics to the system it is possible to take, having a gentle stimulating influence on the whole chain of the endocrine glands. Hence, it is of considerable value in cases of exhaustion and general debility, impotence etc. It also cleanses the blood and gives tone to all organs of the body. The dose is half a teaspoonful of the fluid extract of the bark, or 10 to 15 drops of the fluid extract of the berries, in hot water before meals.

Prickly Ash is usually one of the ingredients in the famous herbal Composition Powder. Has some value in rheumatism and fibrositis.

In homoeopathic potency, when it is known as Xanthoxylum, it covers a wide field, and has proved itself to be a superior remedy for toning up the sensory nerves, bronchial tubes, throat, lungs, nasal membranes, external female organs, testicles, ovaries, pituitary gland, pineal gland, suprarenal glands, thyroid and parathyroid glands. It may be taken for disorders and weakness in any of these glands and organs. We advise four or five pills of Xanthox. 30. on rising and on retiring for three weeks. Debilitated people should give this remedy a trial.

PRIMROSE

The common Primrose (Primula Vulgaris) is not recommended for use as a medicine in the home. It is somewhat poisonous, and some people are very allergic to it. The variety known as Primula Obconica is employed in homoeopathic potency for moist eczema and rheumatism. A dose of four or five pills of Primula Obconica 3, three times daily, has been known to clear up eczema, skin rashes and rheumatism when other remedies have failed. If results are not obtained within two weeks it is wise to abandon the medicine; if progress has been made continue taking for some time. The 30th potency will sometimes clear away patches of brownish pigmentation in the skin, and this has been observed by the writer. Take five pills in the 30th potency on rising and on retiring.

PROSTATE GLAND TROUBLE

A great many men suffer from an enlarged prostate gland, especially after middle age. In our opinion scores of operations for this trouble are unnecessary; unless the condition is too advanced to yield to proper medicinal treatment.

Both the herbal and the homoeopathic schools recommend Saw Palmetto (Sabal Serrulata) berries as being one of the best possible remedies, and there is abundant proof that cures have taken place. The dose of the fluid extract is 10 to 20 drops in a wineglassful of warm water before or after every meal. There is also plenty of evidence that the common fluid extract, although possessing curative virtues, is not to be compared with the fresh plant mother tincture as prepared by homoeopathic chemists. Five to ten drops of this, three times daily, will certainly produce better and quicker results. In our own experience Sabal Serrulata has done some very good work in many prostatic cases.

There are other excellent remedies which can be tried if Sabal Serrulata fails, and all are homoeopathic and harmless. In many instances the following has achieved the most satisfactory results: Take five pills of Thlaspi 30. on rising and again on retiring, and five of Kali Phos. 30. a few minutes before the midday meal. Keep this up for several weeks. A dose of Sabal Serrulata mother tincture may also be taken after meals when on this system; although this is optional.

If the results are very slow try taking a daily dose of Calc. Fluor. 30. in place of the Kali Phos.

Some herbalists advise a poultice of Slippery Elm (without any addition) over the lower part of the abdomen, to be kept on all night. The poultice should be kept in position with a wide bandage; but do not bind too tightly. Powdered Marshmallow may be used in the same manner. A teaspoonful, or a little more, of chloride of potassium may be well mixed with either poultice.

PSYCHOLOGY

It is impossible to discuss fully this vast subject in a book of this size but Psychology plays an important part in the attainment of health and happiness.

People who take an interest in life and the welfare of others, striving to help those who are in need, seldom have to resort to psychological help, they are too busy to allow their troubles to play a major role in their lives.

Feelings of inferiority, of guilt and of mental or spiritual poverty cause maladjustment to life. Illness of mind, or of body, or of both, follow such feelings even as night follows day.

Endeavour to keep busy both mentally and physically as this will help to avoid the necessity of psychological help.

Try this experiment. Stand before a mirror and deliberately look miserable. Can you imagine the face you see inviting happiness? If the same expression is maintained for any length of time you will begin to feel exactly how you appear. Now smile deliberately and the reflection will be entirely different and after a short time you will begin to feel happier! The physical act actually make you feel different and if you make an effort to retain a happy expression you will soon feel the benefit.

By avoiding reading matter that requires thought, a person establishes a habit that prevents creative thinking. The habit tends to encourage mental stagnation and laziness. To read good books slowly is excellent for the nerves and for mental tension.

Remember that homoeopathic medicines can have a profound effect on both mental and physical symptoms and readers are advised, where necessary, to study the remedies mentioned under Mental Remedies with the view of finding a cure.

PSYLLIUM

Psyllium seed is something like Linseed in appearance and virtue. It is used chiefly as an intestinal activator and lubricant. When moistened the seeds swell into a gelatinous mass. They are tasteless, and cause no intestinal discomfort. The dose is two to four teaspoonsful after each meal for adults, and one teaspoonful for young children. Place the seed in a cup and add a wineglassful, more or less, of warm water. Stir until the mixture thickens. Swallow the contents. Or, the mixture may be eaten with soaked prunes for breakfast. Flavour with Lemon or orange juice if desired. Psyllium is most helpful for constipated people with weak or irritable intestines.

PUFF BALL (Bovista)

This is used by homoeopaths. In potency it is one of the best remedies for anaemia, as it has a direct action on the red bone marrow, assisting in the production of red blood cells. It also has a tonic effect on the lungs, pancreas and suprarenal cortex; hence it is of value in general debility and constitutional weakness; also for some cases of irritable coughs. Use the 3rd or 30th potency. If using the 3rd take five pills before meals, three times daily. If the 30th, take five pills on rising and five on retiring, for two or three weeks; longer if necessary. When ordering ask for Bovista.

PULSATILLA

The Pulsatilla, or Wind Flower, is not appreciated as much as it should be by herbalists. It is a superior tonic to the nervous system, the generative organs of both sexes and to the veins. Note, however, that the dose is small: one drop in a little water before meals. No harm will be done if two drops are taken, but neither will better results be achieved. The remedy in potency is recommended, when it covers a very wide field. There is one type of individual, usually female, that responds to Pulsatilla for almost anything that happens to be wrong, from weakness and disordered digestion, to period pains and insomnia. This person is the blond who is inclined to stoutness, easily reduced to tears, upset by taking fats and who is something like an April day in disposition: very changeable. Of course the remedy suits other types, but for this class of person it is a truly remarkable remedy. It acts in almost any potency. We suggest the 3rd. Take four or five pills before meals, three times daily, for stomach upset, nervous dyspepsia, disordered liver, irregular or painful periods, impotency and nervous exhaustion with depression. May also be tried for varicose veins. Has produced some speedy cures in cases of measles and rheumatism, especially the rheumatism of weepy, blond females.

When the 3rd potency fails, try the 30th, when the dose is five pills morning and night for two or three weeks in chronic states. Take every four hours for acute conditions. If correctly selected it acts on acute conditions, such as an upset liver, very quickly.

PUMPKIN

Pumpkin seeds have been used for generations as a worm remedy. They are powerful, harmless and effective. The sufferer fasts for one day during treatment. On rising take a dose of Epsom salts. Prepare the remedy as follows: two ounces of the seeds are beaten up with the same quantity of brown sugar, add milk or water, to make a pint. Divide into three doses. Take one dose one hour after the dose of salts, another at midday and the final dose at 8 p.m. On going to bed take a dose of Castor oil. May be repeated in a week or so if necessary.

PURGATIVES

Unless absolutely essential purgatives should be avoided as they weaken the bowels and eventually produce chronic constipation. When the bowels are very obstinate Senna pod tea may be taken, or a dose of Cascara. It is better to rely on the enema and a laxative breakfast. (See remarks under Constipation).

PYORRHOEA

A treatment that seldom fails is to massage the gums with oil of Eucalyptus at night, and with distilled extract of Witch Hazel in the morning. Or, if you prefer, reverse the order of application and use the Witch Hazel at night. Well rub the insides and outsides of the gums. Keep up the treatment until the condition clears. Compound tincture of Myrrh is also a good application, although Eucalyptus and Witch Hazel are better. See also under **Gums**. Pyorrhoea is due to faulty feeding; also too much mushy food. Give the teeth some exercise and partake of natural foods that require chewing. If the gums are septic take five pills of Baptisia 3. after every meal.

QUASSIA

A tonic to the digestion and a very good worm remedy. Not so long ago cups were turned out of Quassia wood and used as 'tonic makers'. They were filled with water which became charged with the bitter taste of the wood. The water was taken after it had been standing in the cup for some time. These 'tonic makers', or 'bitter cups', are no longer obtainable.

The infusion of one ounce of Quassia chips in one pint of cold water is taken in tablespoonful doses, before or after meals, for loss of appetite, feeble digestion and debility. For worms the dose should be a wineglassful three times daily. Vary the dose for children according to age. Owing to the bitterness most children refuse to take Quassia water, and it should not be forced upon them. Of course it may be flavoured with Liquorice.

QUINSY

An old country remedy is to saturate a large folded handkerchief with oil of Peppermint and bind round the throat (not tightly). The oil is expensive these days, so the essence may be tried. A simple cold water throat pack is also helpful.

A tea made with Sage, taken four or five times daily, is a very satisfactory remedy, the value of which has been proved over and over again.

The homoeopathic treatment which produces speedy and certain results is to take two tablets of Baryta Carb. 6x and five pills of Belladonna 3, alternately. Take the Baryta Carb. at 8 a.m., the Belladonna at 9; the Baryta Carb. at 10 a.m., the Belladonna at 11 a.m., and so on throughout the day until symptoms improve, and then less frequently.

In all cases a gargle of a few drops of the fluid extract or tincture of Hydrastis (Golden Seal) in half a cup of warm water, two or three times daily is helpful and soothing. (See also under **Sore Throat**).

RADIATION

In our explosive modern world the dangers from radiation are on the increase. We are frequently asked if there is a remedy to counteract the effects of radiation. Knowledge is very limited; but we can suggest a remedy which has been used with success in dealing with the effects of radium-therapy on the human body. If this remedy can clear up the bad results of medical radiation with radio-active substances, it seems reasonable to suppose that this same remedy would be helpful to a degree in dealing with radiation in the event of the atmosphere being charged with harmful rays in war, or by accident, in peace. The remedy is a form of radium, so the homoeopathic law of 'like cures like' is brought into play.

Radium Bromide 30. should be ordered from a reliable homoeopathic chemist. Should there be **trustworthy evidence** that one has been subject to radiation, take five pills of Radium Brom. 30. morning and night for one week, and then once daily until all danger has passed. The treatment is harmless, and is the best advice that can be given owing to lack of actual experience — which, for everybody's sake, we hope we shall never have.

Experiments have suggested that lemon and acid fruit juices help to guard against radiation. Bladderwrack (kelp) also seems to have some effect in certain forms of fallout.

RADISH

These tasty vegetables have blood-cleansing properties. Many people like them, but find that they cause indigestion. Eat the green tops with the root and you will probably find that they will agree with you, for nature has so arranged matters that tops and roots taken together supply the factors which enable the stomach to deal with the problem. The Black Radish is a powerful alternative, and has helped to clear up very nasty toxic conditions. Scrape the roots, mash up with a little fresh cream and eat with some of the green tops. It is claimed that Black Radish eaten two or three times daily, will eventually clear the system of all morbid matter. This is doubtful; although great benefit has resulted in the treatment in some serious blood disorders.

RASPBERRY

The leaves of the garden Raspberry are an excellent medicine for pregnant females, giving strength and rendering parturition easy and speedy. This has been proved over and over again, and women who have endured difficult births have been pleased and surprised at the difference experienced at childbirth following a course of Raspberry leaf tea. The tea is also excellent for sore throats and for the stomach complaints of children. May also be used as a gargle when the throat is sore and inflamed. Forms a good wash for sores and ulcers.

Infuse one ounce in a pint of boiling water. Allow to stand for 15 minutes. As a medicine take a cupful three times daily, before or after meals. The tea may also be taken hot during labour, when it is made more potent if a little herbal Composition is added to each dose. For another good medicine containing Raspberry see **Pregnancy.**

RED CLOVER

The flowers of the Red Clover are one of our finest blood cleansers. They are excellent for all blood and skin disorders, morbid and toxic conditions of the system; also for bronchitis and whooping cough. Infuse an ounce in a pint of boiling water; allow to stand for a while and take a wineglassful to a teacupful, according to age, three times daily. For coughs add plenty of Honey and Lemon to make a syrup, and administer a tablespoonful every hour. If the fluid extract is used the dose is a teaspoonful in hot water; or, made into a syrup by mixing one ounce of the extract in a pint of water with enough Honey. Add Lemon if desired. Dose as above.

Freshly gathered Red Clover flowers are excellent for the blood when added to salads. The white blossoms may also be used in this manner, although the red are better. They are perfectly harmless.

RED ROOT

Prepared homoeopathically in the 3rd potency, Red Root (Ceanothus) is an established remedy for anaemia. Many practitioners regard it as being one of the best for this condition. Take four or five pills before meals three times daily.

RED SAGE

This is the common garden Sage. It is one of the best remedies for sore and septic throats, quinsy, laryngitis, tonsillitis and ulceration of the throat and mouth. The Chinese think highly of it, and use it in preference to their own tea. Many housewives make the daily brew with equal parts of Sage and ordinary tea. Prepare in a teapot (not aluminium) in the usual way. For medicinal purposes pour a pint of boiling water on an ounce of the leaves and allow to stand for a few minutes. Keep covered. Dose: a wineglassful every two hours. This infusion may be used for gargling, although the most effective gargle is made by pouring half a pint of hot malt Vinegar, and half a pint of cold water, on an ounce of the leaves. Let stand for a few minutes before using. Gargle as often as is necessary.

REJUVENATION

Eternal youth is probably the oldest dream of mankind; yet, 'dying, thou shalt die', is the shadow that looms ahead from youth onwards. The ancient physicians and alchemists all searched diligently for the secret of life. They recommended preparations of Sulphur, Gold, Antimony, Mercury and other minerals and herbs for removing the causes of old age. Some of their discoveries were really good, and are used to this day; but no remedy discovered by man ever has, or ever can, prolong life beyond a certain period. The fact is that there is no secret fountain of life other than unity with the Godhead.

The length of human life, we may say, is determined very largely by the constitution handed down to us. Dissipation in youth, wrong living, unsuitable food and, above all, wrong thinking will rob anybody of years of useful life; while sensible living, conservation of the life force and right thinking will do much to add to life and make it happy and fruitful. A great deal can be accomplished on the mental plane by reading and applying what has been said on Psychology, Love and other matters in this book; and if the health advice given is only partly carried out benefit is bound to take place physically. Never think yourself into disease; think health, and better health will come. Do not visualize old age, but picture yourself as being vital for many years ahead and growing into what, at heart, you really want to be.

Modern scientists, like the ancient physicians, are still trying to discover methods of rejuvenation, and these range from monkey glands to eating the substance of unborn animals. One may rightly assume that the modern seekers after rejuvenation are no wiser than those of old, and in some respects less competent -- they all fail. That which is dead cannot produce life. Many people die many times before they finally pass away. Why bother about the end? Live one day at a time and make living a full and satisfying occupation. Then it may be said of you, in the words of the Bible, that 'he died old and sated with life'!. As has been pointed out elsewhere, there is no known law limiting life; and we believe that the time will come on this earth when men, under the dominion of the Prince of Peace, will have life abundant.

A Method of Physical Rejuvenation

On rising perform Breathing Exercises, and take a cold or tepid Friction Bath; or a Salt Glow if you can manage it.

Have a breakfast of soaked prunes, cereal such as 'All-Bran' and Molasses to keep the bowels active.

One hour before lunch, tea and dinner take a cup of Raspberry Leaf tea. Take it slowly. This gradually cleanses the stomach, intestines and tissues of the morbid matter responsible for disease and debility. Continue with this medicine for at least three weeks — longer if necessary.

Immediately after each meal of the day take a teaspoonful of the following mixture in a wineglass of hot water:

Fluid extract of Oats	2 ounces.
Fluid extract of Gentian	1 ounce.
Fluid extract of Chamomile	1 ounce.

This medicine may be sweetened if desired. Sip it slowly.

Keep to a sensible diet, and well masticate all food.

Try and have 15 minutes on your back after lunch — longer if possible.

Take a sharp walk at least once daily.

Work in some simple Exercises at a suitable time, but not soon after a meal.

For the first week or so make a Bran Poultice and apply it over the entire abdomen. Keep on all night. The organism will take up the organized mineral matter in the Bran, which will give strength to the system and add to the general tone wherever it is needed.

Above all let your thinking be positive.

This system will usually give new life and energy to anybody who uses his will power to carry it out. Results are truly excellent. We make no claim for originality, as the method is based on the teachings of the old and wise herbal school.

Should you have difficulty in relaxing see under **Relaxation**.

If you cannot manage to do all these things, work in what

you can. Every little helps, and you will be rewarded according to your works.

RELAXATION

Disease and unhappiness are associated with tension. It is difficult to think of any physical disorder being present in a normally relaxed organism. It must be pointed out that the relaxation which is desirable is not weakness of the muscles, prolapse etc. That is not relaxation.

A mind at ease is usually happy and contented, and a mind so blessed will do very much to transfer its contentment and repose to the body which it governs.

In our modern world of hurry, relaxation is becoming more and more difficult. We hurry over meals, we run to catch the bus and life is often a fever of excitement. One difficulty is that any effort to relax of itself tends to produce some tension. Is there any method of inducing relaxation that does not call for real effort? If so, that method is ideal. There is such a method; in fact there are several; to describe a very good one will be sufficient. Remember, however, that no matter how good a system of relaxation may be, a troubled, worried mind will prevent the effects desired, or greatly minimise them. Hence, it is of vital importance to eliminate morbid thinking, worry and destructive emotions in order to obtain the best results from any attempt at relaxation (See **Psychology**, **Spiritual aid** etc.). For all that, it is true that the method to be considered will also help to relax the mind.

Many years ago we contacted Mr. L.E. Eeman. This health scientist evolved a method of relaxation which has proved most effective. It is not just an idea, but is based on long study of the human mind and body and the laws governing the organism. We will not go into the scientific reasons for the method, as the available space must be taken up by describing the practical application of Mr. Eeman's discoveries.

Note that in all cases a few minutes deep breathing should precede the attempt to relax. Lie down and endeavour to let go — imagine yourself sinking into a bed or couch, or collapsing like an old sock. Link your fingers lightly over the upper part of the abdomen, and cross the feet over the ankles — right over left or vice versa. Do not allow the fingers to grip. Keep still. Mentally, think of nothing at all (not an easy task); or, visualize a beautiful scene, a delightful painting, a sunny day, blue skies; or, go over some happy incident in your life.

Another idea is to will that your limbs and organs shall relax. Think of the right leg: it has served you well during the day and deserves a rest; so visualise the muscles relaxing totally. Then turn your attention to the left leg in the same manner. Then, the right hand and arm, and the left hand and arm. Then turn the attention to the abdomen: visualize the intestines, kidneys, stomach settling down to a condition of absolute repose. If you have indigestion, this will often result in the trouble disappearing within a few minutes. Following the abdomen turn the thoughts to the chest, and will that rest shall come to the heart and lungs. Think kindly of your faithful organs, and bless them with good thoughts. Then will that the neck shall relax and, finally, the brain.

The linking up of the fingers and the feet 'polarizes' the body and is the greatest physical contribution of which we know to relaxing the tissues and organs; and this makes the mental attempt at letting go all the easier.

This system is of the greatest value in cases of insomnia, disturbed stomach and bowels, extreme fatigue and even for aches and pains. Do not expect outstanding results at first; although some obtain them within a short time. Keep it up! Very often you will fall asleep after a few minutes. If not, try the method again a little later on. Of this you can be certain: while in this polarized condition your mind and body will receive more benefit than you would derive from fitful sleep. Should you wake up during the night, get out of bed and rouse yourself thoroughly. Then, get back into bed and repeat the Eeman system.

Cases of marked abdominal distress have been greatly relieved and cure hastened by adopting the Eeman method, and people who have not been able to sleep in comfort for years have found repose.

Another line of thought is to think backwards. (See **Insomnia**).

A hot foot bath before retiring is also helpful for relaxing the system.

RHEUMATISM AND FIBROSITIS

In some country districts it was the custom to place a teaspoonful of flowers of Sulphur in each sock or stocking. After removing the hose at night the feet were washed in hot water to which a little bi-carbonate of soda was added. There have been reported cures from this method in cases where it has been persisted with for some time. As has been pointed out elsewhere, the body eliminates a deal of toxic matter from the soles of the feet, and the small quantity of Sulphur that may be absorbed into the system is harmless and has a cleansing action on the blood and tissues. The Sulphur probably encourages acid and toxin elinination.

Burdock herb	½ ounce.
Prickly Ash berries	½ ounce.
Guaiacum chips	½ ounce.
Stinging Nettles	½ ounce.

Simmer in two pints of water, in an iron or enamel pot, for 20 minutes. Strain. Take a large wineglassful before every meal. This herbal tea should be most effective in many cases of rheumatism and fibrositis. If the bowels are costive have a laxative breakfast; and, if necessary, take 10 to 20 drops of the fluid extract of Rhubarb on retiring. Rhubarb is one of the least habit-forming laxatives, and has the advantage of being anti-rheumatic.

The above formula may be taken in the form of equal parts of the fluid extracts, when the dose is half a teaspoonful in hot water. Experience shows that the infusion is the better of the two. There are a large number of herbs useful for rheumatism, many of which are described in these pages. All rehumatic sufferers should pay attention to diet (See **Diet**). A hot Epsom Bath (See **Epsom Salts**) two or three times weekly is very effective. Urine therapy has also produced good results.

There are a great number of reliable homoeopathic remedies, and the selection should be made according to the symptoms. It will pay all sufferers from this distressing ailment to read a good homoeopathic materia medica and repertory for full information. The most used remedies are Poison Oak (Rhus Tox.), Bryonia, Urtica Urens, Colchicum, Formica, Silica and Ledum. When there is swelling Apis Mel. is a good remedy. Any of these remedies may be tried in the 3rd or 30th potency. If there are no marked effects from the low potency try the 30th. When the 3rd is employed take five pills a few minutes before meals, three times daily. The dose for the 30th potency is five pills on rising and again on retiring. When there is no evidence of improvement after, say, three weeks, on a selected remedy, try another. Here are a few helpful indications for remedy selection:

Rhus Tox. Patients requiring this remedy are better for 'limbering up'; better after they have moved about, although movement at first may be painful. Tearing pains. Worse in damp weather. Painful joints. Always worse for cold air. Better for warmth and dry weather.

Bryonia. The sufferer is always worse for movement, and much easier when resting. Joints red and swollen. Better when lying on the painful side or for pressure.

Urtica Urens. Aids the elimination of uric acid, and is indicated for gout. Has been used with success in arthritis. Indicated when the skin is irritable, and rheumatism is alternated with periods of nettlerash. Burning and stinging of the skin.

Colchicum. Rheumatism with great prostration. Internal feeling of coldness. Worse at night. 'Pins and needles' in hands and fingers. Gout. A curious symptom for Colchicum is that the sufferer feels better when stooping.

Formica. A remedy for arthritis and rheumatism. When the stomach, kidneys and nerves are upset, this is usually a good medicine. Stiff and contracted joints, with a feeling of strain in the muscles. The lower extremities are usually the more affected. Pains are sudden and severe. Better for warmth, pressure and massage.

Silica. Seems to suit all cases; may be taken as an additional remedy.

Ledum. Rheumatism usually begins in the feet and travels upwards. In some cases skin affections accompany rheumatism. The sufferer is cold, yet cannot stand the heat of the bed. The small joints are those mostly affected. A good remedy for gout. Sore and tender feet usually call for Ledum. The sufferer is easily exhausted.

Do not take herbal and homoeopathic remedies at the same time. When one method fails, try the others; but give everything a fair chance. Remember to cut sugar out of the diet, and use pure Honey instead. Sweeten beverages with Honey, or Molasses.

Here is another recommended method of treatment: to one pint of water add a teacupful of common table salt and one teaspoonful of Cayenne Pepper. Mix and heat to boiling point. Bathe the affected parts with this hot solution for fifteen minutes or longer; or, apply cloths wrung out in the solution. Over the wet cloths apply towelling to keep in the heat and allow to remain on for an hour or so. When possible repeat three times daily. Remarkable cures in people crippled with rheumatism have been attributed to this method. Very effective when the joints are swollen.

Both oil of Wintergreen and oil of Rosemary have been used with success for rheumatism. The dose is five drops of oil of Wintergreen, or twenty drops of oil of Rosemary in Honey or brown sugar on rising, and again on retiring. Wintergreen oil for massage is also helpful.

Tincture of Iodine has also been used with success. The dose is one drop only in a large wineglassful of cold water on rising and again on retiring. Treatment should be kept up for some time. (See also **Arthritis, Myrrh, Rubbing Oils,** and **Salt**).

RHUBARB

China or Turkey Rhubarb has long been used as a laxative. It also has tonic, astringent and stomachic properties. It has been discovered that it helps to clear some forms of skin rash, especially when associated with rheumatism. Rhubarb has the advantage of giving some tone to the bowels while acting as a laxative. In small doses it will cure diarrhoea. Its use over long periods is not advised.

As a laxative take up to half a level teaspoonful of the powdered root mixed up in Honey or Molasses. For diarrhoea and skin rash the dose should be half a saltspoonful in a little warm Milk or water three or four times daily. The smaller dose also aids digestion. Another way of taking Rhubarb is in the form of Tincture of Rhubarb Co. (from chemists). As a laxative take one or two teaspoonsful in hot water at night. For other purposes half a small teaspoonful in cold or tepid milk or water before meals.

For rashes the remedy often acts better in homoeopathic form: five pills of Rheum 30. on rising and again on retiring; or five of Rheum 3. before meals, three times daily.

RHUS TOX (POISON OAK)

While this remedy may be taken in minute doses in ordinary tincture form, it is not advised for home use. Taken in homoeopathic potency all danger is removed and it no longer acts as a poison. In the 3rd or 30th potency it is one of the best remedies for many rheumatic troubles, and some skin disorders. See the various headings for information regarding doses.

RICKETS

Bone Meal is an excellent food in these cases. Pay every possible attention to Diet, Bathing, Breathing, etc.

Here is a very good medicine:

Fluid extract Gentian	½ ounce.
Fluid extract Vervain	½ ounce.
Fluid extract Chamomile	½ ounce.
Fluid extract Comfrey	1 ounce.
Fluid extract Oats	1½ ounces.

Dose: Half to one teaspoonful, according to age, in hot milk or water before every meal. Sweeten with pure Honey. Older children may take larger doses.

In addition to the above we advise two tablets of Calc. Phos. 3x before meals, and two of Silica 6x after meals, three times daily.

RINGWORM

Painting the actual places with ordinary paraffin will be helpful in many cases. Five to ten minutes after painting with the paraffin apply a little olive oil. This prevents soreness. Some skins are too sensitive for paraffin treatment. In such cases apply oil of Cade two or three times daily. Applications of turpentine have also proved successful. Internally, treat as for **Auto-toxaemia**. Or, give a herbal tea or fluid extract of any of the following: Blue Flag, Burdock, Red Clover, Sarsaparilla. Homoeopathic Sulphur 3x is also a very good remedy. Give an eggspoonful of the trituration (or four

tablets) before each meal. Ringworm points to a constitutional condition, and we strongly recommend that a
homoeopath be consulted.

It must be remembered that some external treatments tend
to be suppressive. The cause is not removed and such
suppression can be harmful. Hence the importance of
constitutional treatment.

Dr John H. Clarke advises local applications of Cod-liver
oil daily. For constitutional treatment he advises homoeopathic Bacillinum 200, a dose of three pills night and
morning once weekly for two or three months.

ROSEMARY

'Rosemary — that's for remembrance'. While Rosemary is
symbolic for remembrance, the original idea may well have
come from the fact that Rosemary tea clears the brain and
brightens the mind. Experienced homoeopaths have also
found that Rosemary in high potency certainly stimulates the
mental processes, and in this form has accomplished much
good in cases of poor concentration and bad memory. Cases
are on record where a few doses of Rosemary 200. have
produced some ideal results in loss of memory. It may be
tried without doing any harm. Take five pills of Rosemary
200. on rising, again on retiring and a final dose on rising the
following morning.

Taken as a tea, or in tincture or homoeopathic form it will
help clear away persistent catarrh, improve the condition of
the scalp and encourage the growth of healthy hair. Oil of
Rosemary is excellent for massaging into the scalp for loss of
hair.

From the botanic standpoint, Rosemary is tonic, astringent, nervine and diaphoretic. It may be taken for nervous
dyspepsia, nervous headache and blood disorders. Place a
small handful of the freshly gathered leaves, or leaves and
flowers, in a jug. Pour on a pint of almost boiling water. Stir,
and cover to keep in the steam. After half an hour a small
cupful of this may be taken two or three times daily for
colds, catarrh, indigestion and nervousness. Also good for
headaches. The same infusion may be used as a hair wash.
For this purpose a little common borax may be added. The
dried herb may be used when the fresh is not obtainable, in

which case use boiling water for the infusion.

Rosemary leaves may be placed in cupboards to keep moths and other creatures away. Rosemary tea, taken at night, is helpful for insomnia. An old country method was to stuff a small pillow with a mixture of Hops and Rosemary to induce restful sleep and calm the nerves. For the various disorders mentioned, the oil of Rosemary may be employed instead of the infusion: one drop in brown sugar or Honey two or three times daily. The infusion is likely to produce better results.

ROSES

A great teacher once said: 'If you have but little room in your garden plant Roses.' This delightful queen of flowers, with its rich perfume, gladdens the heart and adds some beauty to living. Roses also possess medicinal virtues for some eye and skin troubles.* For medicinal purposes, however, we mostly employ the hips. Of recent years Wild Rose hip syrup is much in demand for its high content of vitamin C. The best hip syrup can be easily made at home.*

RUBBING OILS

For Rheumatism, painful joints, neuralgia etc.

Oil Olive	4 ounces
Oil Cajuput	1½ ounces
Oil Cinnamon	1½ ounces
Oil To-tree	1½ ounces
Oil Thyme	½ ounce

In severe cases bathe the part in hot water. Dry and massage in the oil mixture once or twice daily. Mostly hot bathing is not necessary. Do not rub inflamed or swollen joints and tissues.

RUE

Garden Rue is a stimulant, antispasmodic and emmena-gogue. In herbalism it is used chiefly for suppression of the menses. For nervous troubles and hysteria it is of service

* See *Health From the Kitchen*, published by Health Science Press.

when taken in small doses. Infuse an ounce in a pint of boiling water and simmer very gently for ten minutes, keeping the lid on the pot. Strain. For suppressed menses take a wineglassful, warm for preference, before meals three times daily. For hysteria and nervousness the dose is a dessertspoonful, three times daily.

In homoeopathic potency it is a very deeply-acting remedy, and will produce the most satisfactory results in strained muscles and tendons, bruised bones and exhaustion. It also has a favourable action on the organs of vision. Think of Ruta (Rue) as a remedy for spinal pains and weakness, pains in the bones and joints — especially of wrists and ankles — sprains and great weakness generally. Use the 3rd or the 30th potency: 3rd potency five pills before meals. 30th potency five pills morning and night. When exhaustion is the leading symptom take five pills of Ruta 200. on rising and again on retiring and for the following two or three weeks, take a dose of Ruta 30. nightly, on retiring.

RUNNER BEANS

Dr John H. Clarke, in his *Dictionary of Practical Materia Medica* (Homoeopathic), gives some interesting facts about the value of the common Runner Bean (Phaseolus). In homoeopathic form it has been proved to be of immense value over and over again in cases of heart disorders, heart failure, disorders of the prostate gland, punctured wounds and urinary complains. Frank Roberts, M.C., M.N.I.M.H., says that: 'It is not improbable that Phaseolus may one day come into its own and be as well-known as penicillin'. A cut up and crushed fresh runner bean (Pod and all) applied as a cold poultice to any punctured wound, forms one of the finest applications possible. Dr Clarke reports an amazingly quick cure of a wound caused by the prong of a garden fork by this method. A Dr Ramm of Germany, discovered the great value of Runner Beans as a medicine for kidney and bladder trouble. He employed it for over twenty-five years, and the successes he obtained caused him to wonder whether there were any limits to the curative virtues contained in this humble vegetable. Had Dr Ramm concocted a special preparation of Runner Beans, given it an important-sounding name, and had he been commercially minded, he might have been hailed as one of the great benefactors to mankind. Being an honest man he disclosed his findings to his' medical colleagues; but they all thought the remedy to be far too simple — not worthy of further investigation. Maybe, they saw there was no money in it, and that it was a remedy that could be used by the 'ignorant'. For kidney troubles, dropsy and heart disorders associated with urinary weaknesses, there are few remedies to equal Runner Beans. The remedy may be used in homoeopathic form, but in this instance we wish to stress its value in the crude form in which it can be prepared at home. The common Bean is one of the few remedies which, it may be said, acts as well in crude form as it does in potency.

To make a medicine for internal use gather fresh Runner Beans (dried beans are useless). Remove the actual beans (seeds), and slice up the whole of the pods, being sure to include the outer edges. Place two ounces of the sliced pods in four quarts of hot water and simmer very gently for four hours. Keep the lid on the pot, which should not be made of aluminium. Then, strain the liquid through muslin, and put it in a cool place for about eight hours. The boiling should be done in the evening, as the medicine, to be totally effective, **has to be taken the day following.**

In the morning again strain the liquid through fine muslin. Do this carefully to prevent any solids passing through. The dose is a tumblerful every two hours. Make freshly every night, and be sure to follow the directions, and strain the medicine carefully. **Do not take what has been made after 24 hours have elapsed from the time of making (boiling),** as it could cause diarrohea in some cases.

Take for as long a period as necessary. Taken in the manner described it is absolutely harmless. Records exist of this home-made medicine having cured profuse urination, all manner of kidney disease, urinary inflammations, trouble with the urinary passages, stone and gravel, pus in the urine, albuminuria, pancreatic weakness, gout, some heart disorders and valvular troubles, prostatic disorders, bleeding from the urinary organs, the effects of punctured wounds, etc.

People subject to kidney disorders may take this medicine for a week once yearly as a preventative. In rare cases the medicine may cause headaches or diarrhoea, although this is unlikely if the directions are followed. Should headaches result, try homoeopathic Bean medicine, Phaseolus 12.Five pills night and morning for the disorders mentioned. If the reverse happens, and the **homoeopathic** preparation **causes** headaches, it is likely that the crude, home-made liquid will **not** do so.

SABADILLA

An ointment prepared from Sabadilla seeds has long been used for destroying vermin. Prepared homoeopathically, it is one of the outstanding remedies for hay fever. (See under **Hay Fever**). Research has shown that it possesses other properties besides acting on the nasal membranes. Sabadilla is a help to sensitive people who are greatly affected by 'outside influences'. In this connection we not only see why it is so valuable in hay fever, but also why, when taken in high potency, it acts on 'touchy people', enabling them to be less sensitive to other people and circumstances. Sensitives may try five pills of Sabadilla 200. on rising, and five again on retiring, and note the effects. As a rule hay fever cases require the remedy in the 30th potency.

SAFFRON

The flower pistils of Saffron (Crocus Sativus) are used in medicine for female pains, irregular menses, hysteria, nervousness and colds. Pour one pint of boiling water over one teaspoonful of Saffron, and allow to stand for half an hour. Take a tablespoonful before meals. Children less according to age. For colds make the doses larger and take the remedy hot.

Taken homoeopathically it has a wider field of action, and is a good remedy for rages, hysteria, drowsiness, lassitude, heavy feeling in the eyes, feeling as though the eyes were full of smoke, constipation in nervous people, sensation as if something were alive in the abdomen, threatened abortion, uterine haemorrhages, wheezy coughs, colds, weakness in the legs and pains in the ankles and feet. Take four or five pills of Crocus 3. a few minutes before meals, three times daily.

ST. JOHN'S WORT

One of our most valuable herbs. It covers a wider field

than ever dreamed of by the old herbalists, and today
chemists are isolating certain elements in the plant to make
the resultant medicine more acceptable to modern science,
and put more money into the hands of the large chemical
firms!. St. John's Wort, as nature gives it to us, does not need
to be 'messed about'. Modern botanic practitioners and
homoeopaths are loud in their praise of this remarkable
plant. It is tonic, healing, expectorant, diuretic and a
stimulating agent to the vital force.

It is excellent for lung complaints, tissue injuries, nerve
injuries, spinal weakness, kidney trouble, rectal weakness,
throat troubles, weak veins, lymphatic disorders and weak
ligaments.

The fresh flowers infused in Olive oil make a most
soothing and healing application to wounds, sores, swellings
and ulcers. It seems to act very quickly when applied to
injured nerves and lacerations of the fingers. Hypericum (St.
John's Wort) ointment has similar uses, the best being that
obtainable from homoeopathic chemists. For internal use place
an ounce of the herb with flowers in a jug. Pour on one pint
of boiling water, and allow to stand for half an hour. Dose: a
small wineglassful before meals. Children less according to
age. May be given for any of the troubles mentioned above.
For deeply-seated and chronic conditions the homoeopathic
30th. potency is advised. This is especially good for spinal
troubles and internal injuries. Dose: five pills morning and
night.

ST. VITUS' DANCE

Scullcap herb	¼ ounce
Chamomile herb	¼ ounce
Valerian herb	¼ ounce
Liquorice root	¼ ounce

Place in a jug and pour on one pint of hot water. Allow to
stand for an hour. Give a teaspoonful to a tablespoonful,
according to age, a few minutes before meals, three times
daily. Homoeopathic Gelsemium 3. is also a good remedy:
three or four pills after meals. If worms are associated, treat
accordingly.

SALIVA

Believe it or not — your saliva is one of the finest medicines you can take for digestive trouble. As has been stated elsewhere, saliva is a highly organized chemical substance which converts starches into sugar, and prepares the food for the further processing that takes place in the stomach. Hence, the vital importance of thorough mastication. Even if you pay reasonable attention to chewing your food, it may well be that sufficient saliva has not been mixed with it in the mouth. If you masticate imperfectly, then what we have to say is all the more important.

A few minutes before a meal, sit down and work your tongue and cheeks about to encourage the mouth to fill with saliva. Swallow the saliva, and repeat this two or three times. Do the same thing a few minutes after a meal. Should you have symptoms of indigestion, or of flatulence, repeat the process several times; and again a little later if the symptoms persist. A woman of forty years, who suffered badly from acid dyspepsia and marked flatulence from stomach and bowels, cured herself by doing this saliva swallowing over a period of a few weeks. She had been under naturopaths and herbalists for her troubles, with but little relief. Thereafter, she kept her digestion in order by thorough chewing and swallowing her saliva two or three times after meals. An elderly gentleman, who suffered severely from indigestion, and had much pain after nearly every meal, cured himself in the same manner. Indigestion kept another lady awake half the night until saliva swallowing cured her. Suspected duodenal ulceration has also responded to this very simple method. Of course, it is of no value if practiced only for a day or two. Keep it up, and make a habit of it. To be free from indigestion, acidity and pain is well worth the effort. This is another of those very simple things which tend to escape the notice of the learned and scientifically minded. Yet, they know full well that more saliva can and will accomplish such cures.

Saliva has its uses when applied externally. Jesus of Nazareth made clay with his own saliva as an ointment for blindness. Animals always lick their wounds, and we are aware that the chemical composition of saliva is a superior 'medicine' for all sores and wounds. The combination of pytalin with sulpho-cyanate may be the reason. A certain Bridget Bostock, who resided in Cheshire, made it her business during all of her lifetime to treat all manner of diseases by applying her fasting spittle. And, according to the records, her cures were amazing. She used nothing else. Maybe, she was so constituted chemically that her saliva was particularly potent. Bridget cured blindness, deafness, lameness, dropsy, hysteria, falling sickness, leprosy, corns and almost every disease under the sun; but she refused to touch cases of venereal disease. She merely stroked the painful or affected areas with her saliva, and treated her patients while she fasted. It appears that after food has been taken the saliva is less potent. Old Bridget accepted no money or gifts for her cures. It is possible that this strange old lady, who sometimes treated up to seven hundred cases a day, may have possessed some cosmic power which was transferred by means of her saliva; her personal touch may of itself have been sufficient to stir into activity the healing force residing in the bodies of her patients. Mrs. Kingsley Tarpey, a lady of advanced years who lived in London, possessed remarkable gifts of a magnetic nature. Mrs. Tarpey healed by holding the hands of the sufferer for a few minutes, or by applying oil or wool that had been magnetized by her. The writer can testify from first-hand experience as to her powers; and so can many doctors. Investigating scientists regarded her as a sort of cosmic transformer.

The useful properties of saliva are set forth by a physician who lived in 1821. His treatise, now in the British Museum, shows that saliva can cure all the ailments mentioned above. He achieved hundreds of cures by getting his patients to chew a crust of bread until liquified in the mouth, the object being to make the salivary glands liberate a quantity of saliva. The masticated crust was then swallowed while fasting, before breakfast. This daily practice was kept up until the sufferer was well.

We can be sure that, while the astounding cures mentioned may have been due in part to other reasons, nothing but good can result from swallowing one's own saliva, especially while fasting; or, from applying it to sores, wounds, aches and swellings. Use your own saliva and add years of comfort to your life.

SALT

The common salt especially prepared for table use is mixed with chemicals, to make it pour nicely. Shun it! Use plain, untreated salt; or, better still, sea salt, which is sold by chemists for the purpose. There is no doubt that most civilised people take far too much salt with food. If foods were cooked conservatively to retain their natural flavour the call for salt and seasoning would be less. Natural foods have their own salt content. The excessive use of salt causes catarrh, diseases of the mucous membrane and skin troubles. Many writers blame salt for too many troubles, and they go against known facts when they claim that we should not take any salt at all. That is another nature cure illusion. Animals will go for miles in search of salt licks, and unspoilt natives in foreign lands think highly of it.

As salt will cause catarrh, skin and membrane disorders, it follows that, taken in homoeopathic potency, it will cure many of these conditions. In fact, potentised common salt (Natrum Mur) is one of the most powerful remedies in the homoeopathic pharmacopoea. To mention a few: Natrum Mur. is a proved remedy for the ill effects of worry and grief, great weakness and weariness, emaciation (especially noticeable in the neck), anaemia, intermittent fever, hay fever, running colds and catarrh, rheumatic gout, blinding, throbbing headaches, running eyes, cracks and ulceration in the corners of the mouth, cracked lips, suppressed menses, palpitation, back pains and extreme chilliness. As a rule thin, watery catarrh will yield quickly to Natrum Mur.

Four or five pills of Natrum Mur. 12. may be taken night and morning for any of the chronic conditions mentioned. For acute troubles, such as colds, dissolve a dozen pills in half a tumbler of warm water, and take a teaspoonful every two hours for a few doses; and then less frequently.

When a person has many Natrum Mur. symptoms, is thin, weary, scraggy-necked, has watery catarrh and tends to weep easily, this remedy will produce good results in almost any complaint he may have. Such people are advised to take two or three doeses of Natrum Mur. 200. as a 'type medicine': five pills on rising, five on retiring, and a final dose on rising the next morning. Note the results. If the remedy has been well-chosen the effects will be most noticeable over a period of some weeks. The full good effects may take some time to manifest in the system.

To return to salt in its crude form. Moistened salt, applied to burns in time, will usually prevent blistering. Lemon juice with salt is splendid for relieving pain. Heat sufficient salt in the oven, or over a fire, and place it in a flannel bag. Apply the salt bag over the affected area, as hot as can be borne. Cover with a thick towel or blanket and allow to remain for thirty to sixty minutes. Renew if necessary. The hot salt bag is recommended for neuritis, face-ache, sciatica and rheumatic pains in muscles or joints.

The following treatment is said to cure or give much help in cases of rheumatism.

Spread a good layer of common household salt on brown paper, or on newspaper. Whenever convenient relax in a chair with bare feet resting in the salt, and not for less than half an hour at a time, longer if possible. This simple treatment is reported to have done an enormous amount of good in a large number of stubborn cases.

SANDALWOOD

This is a proven remedy for disorders of the mucous membranes, especially of the urinary organs. It is very soothing and healing to the parts. Both the fluid extract of the wood and the oil are used in medicine. The fluid extract is probably the better of the two. Dose: one teaspoonful in warm water before every meal.

SARSAPARILLA

The root of Sarsaparilla is one of the best alteratives known. That is to say, it purifies the blood and eliminates morbid matter from the system. Use for all manner of blood and skin disorders. Also of some value in rheumatism. It is effective in both the fluid extract and homoeopathic form. The dose of the fluid extract is half to one teaspoonful in hot water before or after meals, three times daily. Five pills of Sarsaparilla 3. may be taken if preferred three times daily. Only good can result from this established remedy.

SASSAFRAS

A good remedy for skin disorders, rheumatism and gout.

The root bark is made into a medicine by infusing an ounce in a pint of water, and simmering gently for fifteen minutes. Strain. Dose: a tablespoonful, three times daily. The dose of the fluid extract is half a teaspoonful in hot water. Has some value in catarrh.

SAW PALMETTO

The berries of the Saw Palmetto, or Sabal Serrulata, form one of the finest of remedies for disorders of the prostate gland, wasting of the mammary glands or testicles and most wasting diseases. It increases strength and helps to put on weight. Saw Palmetto seems to have a toning effect on all glandular tissues. It is a natural, nutritive tonic, with diuretic and sedative properties. Unfortunately, the fluid extract of the dried berries has but little value, and the results are nothing to be compared with those obtained by taking the fresh berry tincture. As the berries have to be imported, it is difficult to obtain the fresh plant preparation. Homoeopathic chemists supply it.

A great deal about this remedy has been written by herbalists and homoeopathic physicians. Great stress is placed upon its toning effects on the generative organs, and not enough on its other actions on the endocrine system, nerves and tissues. We have known some bad cases of enlargement of the prostate gland respond to Saw Palmetto; also atrophy of the gland. So we assume that its effect is to normalise tissue. We have also witnessed withered female breasts become normal under its influence.

The dose for the fluid extract is ten to twenty drops in hot water before meals, three times daily. For best results take the fresh tincture, for which the dose may be slightly smaller. While improving the physical defects, this remedy also has a very good influence on the mind — languor, apathy and indifference. A medicine for the weary.

SAWDUST

Yes, there are many uses for discarded sawdust! Properly prepared it makes a wonderful poultice for rheumatism, painful joints, pains in the bones, spinal weakness and lumbago. Also for nerve pains. No doubt if sawdust cost £1.00 per pound it would be highly valued; yet, few common articles surpass this simple item for the purpose mentioned.

All sawdust is good, but the best for making a poultice is from pine wood. We believe that the good comes from the fact that sawdust contains a very large quantity of highly organised mineral matter. The hot sawdust draws the blood to the area treated, and the system absorbs what it requires from the application. Merely scald fresh sawdust with hot water and apply as hot as the sufferer can stand it. The poultice should be large enough to well cover the area affected. Renew in an hour if necessary. Herbs, such as Comfrey, may be mixed with the sawdust. Also, Bran and sawdust make a good mixture.

SCALDS
The information given under **Burns** also applies to scalds. In severe cases seek professional aid.

SCARLET FEVER
As a preventative, when there is a danger of infection, five pills of Belladonna 3. morning and night, are helpful. Two very good remedies for the condition are Belladonna 3. and Baptisia 3.Four or five pills of Belladonna 3. one hour, and the same of Baptisia 3. the next hour; and so on, alternately, for the duration of the disorder. As improvement takes place administer less frequently.

The herbal treatment, if preferred, consists of equal parts of the fluid extracts of Catmint, Chamomile and Scullcap. Dose: a few drops to a teaspoonful, according to age, in hot water every two hours. The bowels are best kept open with warm enemas, with a teaspoonful of the above mixture added. However, it must be stressed that the wise plan when anybody has this form of fever is to seek professional aid. This is most strongly advocated.

SCHROTH CURE
This German method of natural healing, named after its originator, was very popular on the Continent fifty years ago. Indeed, it is still used with great success in some nature cure health homes. The 'Riposo' health home in England is one such establishment, where this method has been used for many years, and is still very popular with the highly efficient

people who run the place. The cure may be the somewhat heroic method employed by Schroth, or a modified and easier system.

The idea is to encourage the elimination of toxic causes and restore the system's vital, healing energy by the withdrawal of food and drink, especially the latter. Under this system the entire digestive system is rested, morbid deposits liberated and the system cleansed of disease-causing substances.

The original very strict system is not a pleasant experience for the sufferer; but the results obtained are often amazing. It is not wise to take the Schroth cure at home, but in an institution where the patient is under expert observation. In such circumstances no harm can be done, and only good result. It has been said that the Schroth system is the cure for the incurable! There is no doubt whatever that the blood is purified and a mass of toxic, disease-causing filth removed from the organism. As a result of this eliminative process the cleansed blood is able to build weakened organs, and restore the normal secretions of vital glands. By the partial deprivation of food and liquid, the stomach and other digestive organs are forced to dissolve the dry food taken by means of their own secretions, and without the assistance of other liquids. The result is that, through the lack of water, the morbid matter is used up and eliminated. The use of certain water treatments during the cure speeds the treatment and hastens the good results. There is no doubt that scores of lives have been saved by this method of treatment, deeply-seated diseases removed and miserable lives made happy. The writer has great faith in the Schroth cure and would undertake it himself if occasion demanded.

SCIATICA

The treatment given for **Rheumatism** will often cure the worst cases of sciatica. There are, however, instances where skilled manipulation of the hip and lower spine, massage, heat treatment or packs or poultices are essential. Try the herbal medicine advised for Rheumatism and apply hot Bran, Mustard, Chamomile or Sawdust poultices. These should be applied to the small of the back. Use large poultices — small ones are useless.

One old method was to heat a flat iron, and then cover the iron with woollen material well moistened with Vinegar. Apply over the buttock, and also down the thigh over the painful area. Do this two or three times daily. The heat should be as much as the sufferer can bear.

Homoeopathic treatment for this painful condition can be most effective. We have known cases, even of aged people, respond to this treatment: five pills of Colocynth 3. before meals, and five of Colchicum 3. after meals, three times daily. Other cases respond to five pills of Rhus Tox., three times daily. Those interested in the Schuessler system of bio-chemistry may dissolve about ten tablets each of Kali Phos. 6x and Mag. Phos. 6x in half a tumbler of hot water, and sip a dessertspoonful every hour when pain is severe; or, every two hours as the condition improves.

Sufferers should keep the affected leg raised on a chair during the day, and on a pillow when in bed.

SCULLCAP

One of the best nervines in the botanic materia medica. It is also a tonic and is strongly antispasmodic. It has been used for generations as a successful medicine for hysteria, neuras-thenia, insomnia, nerve pains, rickets, St. Vitus' dance and wherever nervous trouble exists in the body. It is absolutely harmless. Simmer one ounce in a pint of water, using an iron or enamel pot, for ten to fifteen minutes. Simmer gently, and keep the lid on the pot. Strain. Dose: a wineglassful every hour in cases of hysteria and nerve pains. For general purposes take 3 times daily, before meals. Children less according to age. May be sweetened with Honey or slightly flavoured with Liquorice. Dose for the fluid extract: half a teaspoonful in hot water, as above. The extract is not so effective as the infusion.

SEA SICKNESS

During an attack of sea or travel sickness take a cup of *hot* water at ten to fifteen minute intervals. This simple method will usually produce speedy ease. To prevent this form of sickness be careful what you eat before departing on your journey. Let the food be light, and have the juice of a large lemon with a pinch of common salt in it a few minutes before you start. A little lemon taken at the first sign of sickness will also prove most helpful. There are some effective homoeopathic remedies which can be taken as preventatives, and they may be taken in combination. Go to a homoeopathic chemist and get a mixture in liquid form of equal parts of Cocculus 30., Tabacum 30. and Petroleum 30. Take five drops in a dry spoon half an hour before the journey, five immediately before starting and five a little later on. This will usually prevent all sickness. May also be taken during the journey, should it be necessary.

The following, by F. J. Mortimer, appeared in *The Listener*: 'Let me tell you how photography can be turned to account as a cure for seasickness. Take your camera with you. Have a direct-vision view-finder, through which you boldly look at the scene that you are going to photograph. Such a view-finder can easily be fitted to any camera, even those of the reflex type. The plain wire frame kind is best. Then, at intervals, when things get dangerous, keep your eye at the view-finder, and sight the skyline through it, as though about to take a photograph. Your body will automatically adjust itself to the movement of the boat, the eyes are occupied, the mind concentrated — and you won't feel sick.'

SELF-PITY

Self-pity is a mental disease; for how can one be 'at ease' when feeling sorry for oneself?. To be ill at ease is a form of disease. Those who suffer from this very common mental state should read the information given under **Psychology, Spiritual Aid, Love**, etc. See also under **Mental Remedies**.

SENNA

Many adults will shudder at the very mention of Senna tea. When the writer was a child he recalls being violently sick after a swallow of the brew; but in those days, for some reason, the tea was made from the leaves of the plant, now the pods are used. A tea made from Senna pods is not unpleasant, and is not to be compared with the awful brew forced upon us when we were children with the object of giving the bowels a good clear-out. The pods are sold by all herbal vendors and chemists, with instructions on the carton. The strength of the infusion depends on age and the state of the bowels. Senna is harmless; but, as with all purging medicine, it should only be taken when necessary. The fluid extract may be used instead of pod tea, when the dose varies from an eggspoonful to a teaspoonful in warm water, flavoured with Honey and/or Liquorice if desired,

A teaspoonful of Senna pod tea, or two drops of the fluid extract in a little water, taken before meals, is a suitable medicine for the colic and flatulence of young children.

SEX TROUBLES

Helpful information is given under **Female Troubles, Impotency** and **Marriage.**

SHINGLES

Nettle tea has proved very effective for shingles; but the method which has brought us the greatest success has been homoeopathic. No doubt straight homoeopaths can select the one single remedy which meets the requirements of each individual case. Our method has been to administer a series of remedies. Results are produced, so why worry over finding one remedy out of a large number? After all, shingles cause much distress, and prompt action is called for. Here is the method we have adopted with marked success.

On rising, five pills of Titanium 30.

Before lunch and the evening meal, five pills of Formica 30.

After lunch and the evening meal, five pills of Rhus Tox. 30.

Cease taking the remedies as soon as the symptoms depart.

Cloths wrung out in equal parts of cold water and Vinegar may be applied frequently to painful areas. If this seems to cause extra irritation, use rather less Vinegar and more water. Or, sponge the areas with Vinegar and water. Gentle massage with Olive oil suits some people better.

SINGING

Singing is a grand exercise for mind and body. It improves the lung capacity, activates the digestion and aids the circulation. At the same time it helps to take the mind off morbid thoughts and reduces tension. Singing helps one to be happy, and those who cannot sing with melody can at least make a joyful noise. King David knew of the value of song, and there is sweet music in his psalms. Singing has always been associated with happiness, both here on earth and with the hosts of heaven. When the earth was formed the morning stars sang together for joy. We read of the song of Moses and the Lamb, and of the singing of a new song when Paradise has been restored on earth.

When feeling low, pull your shoulders back and SING! Singing will do much to change your line of thought, and the effort will do good in more ways than one. When circumstances permit, sing as you work. Native people realise the value of song in their work. It puts rhythm into movement and enables one to do things better, and sometimes, quicker.

It is possible to make living a melody — a harmony, a song. One helpful way of making living a harmonious process is to sing whenver you can.

SKIN DISEASES

See under the various headings, **Acne**, **Eczema**, **Irritation** etc.

SKUNK CABBAGE

This is a harmless anti-spasmodic, and is of much value in most spasmodic conditions and where tension exists. Advised for asthma, stomach and abdominal pains and for nerve pains and flatulence.

Take about half a teaspoonful of the fluid extract in a little hot water before or after meals, or as required. May be sweetened with honey or brown sugar.

SLIPPERY ELM

The powdered bark of the Slippery Elm (Ulmus Fulva) tree forms one of the finest healing foods known. It is as nourishing as oatmeal, is soothing and healing to the mucous membranes and is very easy to digest and assimilate. Hence, it is of great value in gastric disorders, stomach and duodenal ulcers and inflamed states of the intestines. Moreover, its healing virtues are carried to other organs in need of soothing treatment. Here we have the ideal combination of good food and potent medicine. There are several reliable Slippery Elm foods on the market, although the actual Elm content is not very much. Wheaten or other cereal flours and various substances are added to make bulk; and this is quite in order. We would, however, point out that although wholemeal flour is regarded with favour, coarse wholemeal flour is not advisable with Slippery Elm in cases of ulceration, for the Bran tends to irritate and take away some of the value of the Elm. In our opinion Slippery Elm foods with Maize, Barley, Arrowroot, Comfrey and other foods free from irritants are more helfpul in such cases.

Slippery Elm is difficult to mix, although mixing is easier when it is blended with other ingredients. When using plain Slipper Elm place a teaspoonful in a cup, add an equal part of brown sugar or Honey and mix. Then add a very little cold water and again mix thoroughly. Gradually fill up the cup with hot milk, water, or half milk and water and continue to stir vigorously. This is a nourishing, healing meal; and, when the sufferer is not very hungry, it is quite unnecessary to take any other food. In severe cases of gastric distress, ulceration, etc., a cup of this food may be taken four or five times daily for a few days, when, in a large number of cases, the trouble will have disappeared. The food may, if desired, be flavoured with orange juice, prune juice or anything of that nature. When diarrhoea is present prepare as above, but add a teaspoonful of Arrowroot before mixing with cold water.

What this healing food-remedy does internally it also accomplishes externally when the coarse powder is used a a hot poultice for ulcers, wounds, boils, burns, skin disorders and all inflamed surfaces. May be mixed with water or milk for this purpose. It does not suppress. It aids nature in throwing off poisons and morbid matter. For the purposes mentioned there is probably nothing to equal Slippery Elm, and 'worth its weight in gold' is a term that can be truly applied to this wonderful product of the vegetable kingdom.

The remedy can be used as an infusion made from pieces of cut bark, but this is not so effective as the powder. Merely pour boiling water over a few pieces of the bark and allow to stand for fifteen to thirty minutes. Take a cupful as often as desired.

SMOKING

Billy Bray, an old West countryman, used to say that if

God had intended man to smoke an outlet for the smoke would have been provided at the top of his head.

Frankly, it is a bad and dirty habit, and it is a pity that the noxious weed was ever discovered. There is no doubt that it is a contributing factor in lung cancer, catarrh and many respiratory troubles. Young people who start smoking are liable to have lung cancer by the time they reach forty-five to fifty-five years of age. The exceptions are those who smoke moderately and do not inhale. Smoking dulls the mind, poisons the blood, ruins the nerves and reduces the life-span.

We believe that all who really want to stop smoking can do so. The trouble is they do not WANT to. It takes only a little willpower. When the desire comes do something quickly — anything to take the mind off the subject. One method supposed to be successful is to look at the cigarette, say — as though talking to a person — 'I hate you; you are filthy and disgusting'. Then smoke as usual. After doing this for some time the impression of the auto-suggestion of hatred for cigarettes has its effect, and the physical side actually wants to reject the habit.

Some find relief when the desire comes by chewing gum, or sucking a sweet. One man we knew kept a date stone in his mouth. The fact remains that if you really wish to stop smoking you can do so without any aids. Homoeopathic Staphisagria 30. on rising and again on retiring is said to help one overcome the tobacco habit.

SOAP

Ordinary soap is not good for people with sensitive skins, and many of the highly-priced toilet and medicated soaps are not any better. As a rule soaps containing Olive oil are very mild. Herbal soaps (Marshmallow and Slippery Elm are good examples) are advisable. One of the best soaps obtainable is M'Clinton's Colleen. Originally this soap was made with plant ash and was free from soda. Professor Kirk of Edinburgh thought highly of it, and advised it for making soap packs, for massage and various other purposes. We do not know if the quality of this soap is as it was years ago. It is difficult to obtain, and usually has to be ordered from Ireland. Local chemists can obtain it on request.

SOFT WATER

As toxaemia (poisoning — impurities in the system) is a basic cause for so many diseases, it is interesting to note that such a simple item as pure water may be used to free the system of accumulated morbid matter and restore a goodly measure of health. Ordinary tap water should not be used for this purpose, especially if the water has been chlorinated. The water is best when soft or distilled. Use either filtered rain water, or water that has been distilled. Distilled water can be obtained quite cheaply from a chemist's shop; or, one may purchase a small still from an ironmonger. Note, however, that there are certain regulations pertaining to the possession of home stills.

There is no hard and fast rule as to how the soft water treatment may be taken. The water may be used hot or cold, but always it is better taken slowly. When the liver is at fault it is probably better taken hot. The following system is advised for the majority of cases.

On rising: two tumblers.
Mid-morning: two tumblers.
Mid-afternoon: two tumblers.
Before the evening meal: two tumblers.
Before retiring: two tumblers.

This may seem to be a lot of water, but remember that it is a special treatment. It should be continued for at least three weeks, and in marked cases of toxaemia and blood disorders for up to six weeks. Apart from sensible feeding there is no call for special foods, although it is usual for the one taking the treatment to require less food than usual. This is to be expected. Further aid may be accomplished by taking Agar-Agar or Irish Moss tea before retiring.

Very soon the skin becomes clearer, the eyes brighter, the individual more relaxed and general organic function improved. The thin will put on some weight, and the corpulent lose some. By this method the blood and tissues are thoroughly 'washed', and this makes for better nutrition and improved function of all glands and organs.

When distilled water is not possible, use rain water. And, if no filter is available, boil it for ten minutes; pour into another pot (not aluminium); boil again for ten minutes;

repeat the boiling for a third time, allowing the water to cool off before each re-boiling.

The soft water cure will brighten the mind and prove to be of great value in the treatment of indigestion, stomach and duodenal ulcers, nervous troubles and general debility. It is important, however, to point out that sufferers from heart disease, high blood pressure and the more serious kidney disorders should not take this treatment unless under expert supervision.

SORE THROAT

Sage tea is as good as anything the herbal world can offer for sore throats. Take a cup three or four times daily, and also use it as a gargle. A good pinch of powdered Cinnamon may be added. Lemon and Honey also form a good throat medicine. Tincture of Golden Seal makes an excellent throat spray. Just spray the throat with it occasionally.

Among the homoeopathic remedies we have Belladonna 3. and Phytolacca 3. As a rule the former is very effective. Take five pills every hour until the throat is easier, and then less frequently. For the treatment of Quinsy see under that heading. Cold packs to the neck are useful (see **Bathing**). A pack made with equal parts of Vinegar and water is advocated. One may remain on all night; but do not apply tightly.

A popular method of treating sore throat in some country districts is to paint the internal throat with ordinary paraffin three or four times daily. Use a small, soft brush; or, a feather may be used for the purpose.

An ancient remedy was to toast a thick slice of bread, soak it in very hot Vinegar, squeeze out excess moisture, wrap the toast in linen and apply to the throat. Apply as hot as can be borne. This method is claimed to have cured diphtheria very quickly. Repeat the treatment in a few hours time if necessary. A toast poultice may remain on all night. Inhaling the fumes from heated vinegar is also helpful.

SOUTHERNWOOD

An established remedy for obstructed menses which is harmless and effective. The infusion of one ounce to a pint of boiling water is taken in wineglassful doses, three times daily.

Another use for Southernwood is that of a scalp and hair wash. It cleanses and stimulates the scalp circulation, encouraging the growth of new hair. It may be used alone or combined with Rosemary. The combination produces the best results. Infuse half an ounce of each in a pint of hot water. Allow to stand for a few minutes and then well massage the scalp with the infusion. Wash the head first of all. Do this twice weekly. Powdered Southernwood herb is sometimes employed for worms in children. Up to a teaspoonful of the powder is mixed with black treacle or Honey and given night and morning. Repeat in a day or two if necessary.

SPASMODIC TROUBLES

Spasmodic troubles are in the nature of cramps, colic, nervous pain due to tension and contracting of the muscles. To keep a harmless remedy handy for emergencies is very wise, and here is a recipe for Anti-spasmodic drops.

Tinct. of Scullcap	1 ounce
Tinct. American Valerian	1 ounce
Tinct. Myrrh	½ ounce
Tinct. Lobelia seed	½ ounce
Tinct. Wild Yam	½ ounce
Tinct. Capsicum (Cayenne)	½ ounce

Dose: ten to sixty drops, according to age and severity of symptoms, in hot, sweetened water every fifteen minutes. Take much less frequently as the condition improves. If vomiting takes place this is all to the good; although it is unlikely. A dose taken three times daily will help to free the system of impurities and impart strength to the entire organism. Continue for several days. Anti-spasmodic drops are a very good application for nerve pains, sciatica, neuritis, rheumatic pains, etc. Rub in warm, or, apply as a compress.

SPEARMINT

Members of the Mint family are very good carminatives, digestives and blood cleansers, and the common Spearmint is no exception. When in season add fresh leaves of Spearmint to salads and cooked food; also place in sandwiches.

As a medicine, infuse a handful of Mint in a pint of hot

(not boiling) water, and allow to stand for half an hour. A tablespoonful to a wineglassful before meals will aid digestion and help to prevent flatulence. Sweetened, and given in small doses, it is very good for the flatulence and stomach upsets of children.

A leaf of Spearmint, held on the tongue, will prove very refreshing when one is tired and weary.

SPIRITUAL AID

The writer being of the Christian faith approaches this subject from that angle. Those who do not believe in anything beyond what their eyes can see may not wish to read these lines.

There is much evidence of the efficacy of Spiritual Healing but in order to receive divine help it is essential for the sufferer believe in the love of God.

By acceptance of discomfort and pain, of disappointment, misfortune and sorrow, we survive the supreme test of submission to the will of God. In such a state we achieve inward peace and the amazing thing is that once we have arrived at this point a large proportion of the pain and trials, both mental and physical, seem to vanish! In some cases they cease to exist. Faith can remove enormous obstacles; works can achieve the seemingly impossible; faith plus works can perform miracles.

Those seeking Spiritual Aid should strive to live in the spirit of Christ — every minute of every day. The lessons of humility, *selflessness*, and love must be learned.

A most difficult lesson is to learn to love all humanity, both good and bad, but one should remember that everyone is a son of God and there is good in the worst and bad in the best of us.

Prayers should be offered in the spirit of humility, in this respect many people seem to believe that prayers should only be offered for help to achieve their selfish aims, often at the expense of their fellow men! And they blame God when their requests are not answered! 'The humble shall inherit the earth'.

The prayer of St. Francis is as follows. 'Lord, make me an instrument of Thy peace. Where there is hatred, let me sow love; where there is injury, pardon; where there is doubt,

faith; where there is despair, hope; where there is darkness,
light; where there is sadness, joy. O, Divine Master, grant that
I may not so much seek to be consoled as to console; to be
understood, as to understand; to be loved, as to love; for it is
in giving that we receive, it is in pardoning that we are
pardoned'.

SPLINTERS AND THORNS IN FLESH

Homoeopaths advise two tablets of Silica 6x every three
hours to hasten the expulsion of splinters etc.

In stubborn cases a simple hot bread poultice will often
remove the splinter etc.

A very effective method is to obtain a narrow-necked
bottle, fill with hot water and empty when the bottle is really
hot then place the neck opening over the splinter or thorn.
As the bottle cools a vacuum is created, thus drawing the
object to the surface of the skin. This process may have to be
repeated several times, but it rarely fails. It is essential to
press the opening of the bottle hard onto the area to prevent
air entering. This simple method has been employed by
hedgecutters for generations.

SQUILL

This is still a popular ingredient in cough medicines, as it
has been for a very long time. Also has a reputation as a
remedy for simple dropsy, catarrh and asthma. It should
always be administered in small doses. Five drops of the
tincture in warm, sweetened water, three times daily; or, half
a teaspoonful of the syrup of Squill.

STAVESACRE

Used as a medicine for worms, and as an ointment for
vermin. It is not advised by us as a medicine for internal use,
as there are other and better harmless worm medicines.
However, this powerful agent becomes a first rate and totally
harmless healer in homoeopathic form. We have employed it
with marked success in the treatment of impotency, and for
those who have abused their sexual life. For this purpose it
has few equals. The suggested dose is four or five pills of
Staphisagria (Stavesacre) 30. morning and night for three
weeks. If improvement has taken place, cease the remedy for

a week, and then take another course. If there is no improvement, try other remedies.

STINGS (see INSECT BITES)

STONE (URINARY)

This painful condition can often be relieved and cured by simple herbs.

Brew half an ounce each of Barberry Rootbark, Pareira Root, Parsley Herb and Uva-Ursi in two pints of water for about fifteen minutes and strain. Take a wineglassful before meals, three times daily.

In many cases better and quicker results may be obtained by taking the above mixture in homoeopathic form. Obtain the mixture in liquid form comprising equal parts of Berberis Vulgaris, Pareira, Petroselinum and Uva-Ursi in the 3rd potency. Dose is 5 drops on rising and on retiring. It is usually necessary to take the medicine for some time.

STONE ROOT

One of the best remedies for gravel and stone. Take twenty to thirty drops of the liquid extract in warm water before meals, three times daily. In homoeopathic form, when it is known as Collinsonia, it is a great pile remedy. Dose: five pills of Collinsonia 3. before meals; or, five pills of the 30th. potency morning and night for several weeks.

STYE

Belladonna 3. and Pulsatilla 3. in alternation, hourly. Belladonna one hour, Pulsatilla the next, and so on. If suppuration takes place cease these remedies and give Hepar Sulph. 6x trituration — a saltspoonful every two hours. As with most homoeopathic remedies the dose for the Belladonna and Pulsatilla is four or five pills.

SUGAR

White sugar is a denatured commercial product which, although sweet to the taste, is one of the chief causes of an acid constitution. One writer describes commercial sugar as 'the curse of civilization'. That is rather strong language; but white sugar *is* one of our curses. The effects of sugar range from decayed teeth to nervous disorders and rheumatism. Certainly all rheumatic sufferers should avoid it. Sweet fruits are in order, for the sugar in fruits is natural and good. Common moist brown sugar is better than white, but even that is not by any means an ideal sweetening agent. Pure Honey is the best substitute for sugar. (See **Honey**).

SUGGESTION

We live in a world of suggestion. We are hypnotised daily by newspaper advertisements, radio announcements and what is handed out on the T.V. screen. Every display in a shop window is a suggestion that we want this and that, whether we can afford it or not. Advertising is a fine art, and much attention is given by experts on how best to convince people that they just cannot do without certain products. Of course many advertised products are good, and we take off our hats to those who advertise truthfully. The point is that the human mind is always open to suggestion, and if you look at an advertisement long enough, or listen to a voice telling of the qualities and virtues of some product, the idea sinks in that you cannot do without it; and out comes the purse.

We cannot avoid suggestion, but we can be wise and listen to what is sensible and use our own judgment. In the affairs of home life suggestion can be either good or bad. Suggest to a child that he is wicked or useless, and the idea will sink into his mind, and he may become wicked or useless. Give him help and legitimate praise, and he will tend to fashion himself after the image you have implanted in his mind.

Self-suggestion (auto-suggestion) plays a very important part in the lives of all of us. Many suggest illness to themselves until the illness take root, and what has been feared comes about. We have seen this happen over and over again. Likewise, suggest health to yourself, and believe that within you is the power which will enable you to get better, every day and in every way, and you will invite what you visualize in your mind. Of course you must keep to natural law and do your part, and then you will have the good feeling of having earned what you enjoy. A very great help is to suggest to oneself that one has the necessary spiritual aid that comes when a heart is fixed on righteousness (rightness). If, in faith, you seek the aid that is promised, that aid will surely come. If you lack the faith that you will receive help you have no right to expect it; but with the necessary faith, every time you ask for what you need that which is *necessary* will come to you; also you will be constantly suggesting health and happiness to your own being. Faith transforms the mind from negative to positive thinking.

A great deal of wrong information has been written concerning auto-suggestion. It is wrong and harmful to suggest to yourself that you have no pain if pain exists. Such a form of suggestion amounts to suppressive mental dope; and it suppresses just as much as any poisonous drug. We are well aware that the Christian Scientists wriggle out of it by saying that God alone is reality, that pain does not exist as a result, and so forth. We have yet to hear of any person holding this belief prostrating themselves on a railway line before an on-coming train in the belief that the train does not exist. We are here on earth in physical form and must face physical facts. We are here to become in matter what we are in spirit; but that end cannot be attained by living in a realm of imagination. It is the divine purpose that we become physical expressions of the spiritual Creator. We can do this only by keeping to the Creator's laws, with the help guaranteed through Christ. If God intended us to live in a world of spiritual substance we would never have been here on earth. Matter, of course, is crystallised spirit's mortal name; but it is stupid to confuse the two planes of being; they are separate and distinct.

SUMBUL

Sumbul, also known as Musk Root, is an antispasmodic, nerve stimulant and tonic. It is a useful remedy for nervous complaints, over-sensitiveness, low types of fever, asthma and bronchitis. Of great value for hysterical females. The dose is ten to fifteen drops of the fluid extract in a little hot water before meals, three times daily.

Personally, we have found it to be one of the best possible remedies in homoeopathic potency for high blood pressure when due more to mental/emotional causes than to arterial disease; although it has some value in the latter. We give five pills of Sumbul 30. on rising and on retiring for three or four weeks.

SUNDEW

Sundew (Drosera) acts on the respiratory organs and their membranes. It may be employed in material or homoeopathic doses. The dose of the fluid extract for tickling coughs, whooping cough, dry coughs and asthma is ten drops in a little hot water three or four times daily. May be flavoured if desired. The fresh juice has been used successfully as a local application for warts and corns. There is ample evidence that, as an internal medicine, it acts better in homoeopathic form. For any of the complaints mentioned the dose is four or five pills of Drosera 3., three times daily. In chronic conditions use the 30th. potency: five pills morning and night for three or four weeks. Homoeopaths regard it as a specific for whooping cough. It also acts as a prophylactic for this distressing complaint.

SUNSTROKE

Give either Glonoine, Belladonna or Hyoscyamus every hour until better, and then much less frequently until well. We suggest that Glonoine be given in the 12th. or 30th. potency; the other remedies in the 3rd. Do not give all three. Any one will prove most helpful. Additionally, two tablets of Nat. Mur. 30. should be given night and morning for a week or so. Scullcap tea is also good for cases of sunstroke.

SYCOSIS (BARBER'S ITCH)

Treat as for **Auto-toxaemia.** Some cases are very stubborn, and for such we recommend five pills of Psorinum 200. on rising and again on retiring. Just the two doses. If the condition improves, but does not entirely disappear, repeat the two doses in three weeks time. Should there be failure from this treatment, try Thuja 200. Two doses, as for Psorinum. The day following start taking five pills of Thuja 30. morning and night for two or three weeks. Our method of giving homoeopathic medicines differs from that of most homoeopathic physicians; but we are concerned with results and not with methods and ideas, and all the advice given is based on long experience.

TANSY

A successful country herbalist used to give Tansy to almost all his female patients with monthly period troubles.

Among the plant remedies for obstructed menses, generative organ pains and nervous troubles associated with these conditions, we doubt if there exists a better remedy. It is often given with Pennyroyal in equal parts. Tansy will also expel worms in children, when the dose is a small cupful of the tea, sweetened, on retiring and before breakfast. Repeat if necessary. Women with period trouble should take a wineglassful before meals, three times daily for several weeks. The strong tea is not recommended for pregnant females. The infusion is made by pouring a pint of boiling water over an ounce of the herb. Cover, and allow to stand for about half an hour. Better taken hot.

TEA

Weak tea, freshly made, is not as poor a beverage as many writers make out. It is slightly stimulating and very refreshing. It is better flavoured with Honey and Lemon, for which a taste can easily be acquired. Strong tea, and tea that has been left standing for some time, is harmful. It literally tans the stomach and is a cause of much dyspepsia.

A good health tea can be made by using two parts of Indian or China tea with one part each of Red Sage and Lime flowers. Prepare in a teapot in the usual manner. Somewhat more of this mixture is likely to be required than as is the case with ordinary tea. Maté tea is a health giving beverage.

TEETHING TROUBLES

If the mother has lived wisely and dieted sensibly during pregnancy, the child is unlikely to have teething troubles. (See Pregnancy). Should teething be difficult, and there be stomach upset and irritability, the following natural medicine is advised: dissolve four tablets each of Calc. Phos. 3x and Nat. Phos. 3x in a tablespoonful of hot water. Then add ten drops of Chamomilla 1x. Stir. Give the child a teaspoonful of this three or four times daily; or, add it to feeds when bottle fed. This should ensure the growth of healthy teeth and a comfortable stomach. After teeth have formed, should there be any signs of early decay, give two tablets of Calc. Fluor. 6x on rising and two of Silica 8x on retiring, for a few weeks.

TENSION

Read what has been said under the headings of **Peace, Psychology, Relaxation** and **Spiritual Aid**.

There is healing in quietness. *Be quiet* and help will surely come. It is during rest that our problems are solved. Seek quiet places, when possible, where time moves softly on unhurried feet.

Here is a medicine which is soothing to the nerves and has a tranquilizing effect on the mind.

Fluid extract of:-

Passion Flowers	½ ounce
Scullcap	½ ounce
Valerian	½ ounce
Sambul	½ ounce

Dose: a small teaspoonful in a little warm water before meals three times daily. Take another dose on retiring if necessary.

The author's book *Tranquilization with Harmless Herbs* is extremely helpful.

THROAT OBSTRUCTION

A fish bone in the throat can usually be removed by inducing vomiting. Put the forefinger to the back of the tongue to induce this, or take an emetic. To swallow a fairly large piece of bread will often be effective. Drinking slightly diluted lemon juice is another effective method; even to drink several glasses of water will remove small throat obstructions.

Never panic as fear causes tension and adds to the discomfort.

When simple means are ineffective seek professional aid.

THROMBOSIS

May be treated by the same methods as for **High Blood Pressure**. In all cases attention must be given to diet and fried foods and cooked animal fats avoided.

The two leading homoeopathic remedies for preventing and helping to disperse blood clots are Cholesterin 30 and Lachesis 30. Take five pills of the first mentioned on rising and five pills of the latter on retiring for two or three weeks. These remedies may be repeated later if necessary.

Nettle tea may be taken at all times as it will not interfere with the homoeopathic remedies. It is, however, better not taken at the same hour as these remedies.

THUJA

This is the Arbor Vitae, or Tree of Life. Used chiefly by the herbal school for fevers, coughs, gout and amenorrhoea, and in days gone by as a remedy for growths. The homoeopaths have brought this remedy to the fore by their discovery that it is an anti-sycotic of great power, especially when administered in homoeopathic potency. It is given internally for warts, polypi and fleshy excrescences. It acts on the blood, skin, gastro-intestinal tract, kidneys, spinal cord and brain, and is a fine remedy for the ill-effects of vaccination, exhaustion and emaciation. The use of Thuja in potency by skilled practitioners has undoubtedly saved many lives. The laws covering what one may write about concerning remedies prevents a discussion on all the great merits of Thuja. For the layman we recommend five pills of Thuja 30. morning and night for the treatment of warts, polypi, toxaemia and the ill-effects of old toxic states. For infants who never seem well after vaccination, give three drops of Thuja 30. every other day for six doses.

Obstinate catarrh and leucorrhoea will often respond to Thuja when other remedies fail. The strong mother tincture may be applied to warts locally, two or three times daily.

THYME

Both the wild and garden Thyme are useful and effective medicines for flatulent indigestion, convulsive coughs, whooping cough, catarrh and sore throats. Pour a pint of boiling water on an ounce of the herb; cover and allow to stand for half an hour. Dose: a dessertspoonful to a tablespoonful three or four times daily. May be flavoured with Honey or Liquorice to taste. Can also be added to Linseed tea. Give smaller doses to young children.

TOLU BALSAM

The balsam is used in medicines for coughs and catarrhal colds, and has an established reputation. Usually employed in the form of a syrup, it can be obtained from most chemists.

The dose varies from a few drops to a teaspoonful, according to age, three or four times daily. A reliable medicine for chest and lung troubles.

TONGUE INDICATIONS

In spite of recent criticisms about the old method of diagnosing certain conditions of the digestive and assimilative organs from the state and coating of the tongue, we have to go by the exhaustive experience of thousands of doctors and healers, and claim that the tongue gives positive indications which are a most valuable guide in diagnosis and remedy selection.

A bluish-black coating suggests bowel toxaemia.

Brown at the centre, or all over the tongue, indicates bowel trouble, and probably nervous debility.

A dark streak down the centre is another indication of toxaemia, and is often present in cases of typhoid.

A flabby, moist tongue, with imprints of the teeth shows general digestive upset and, very probably, faulty digestive secretions.

When the tongue is furred this points to sluggish digestion, liver upset and acidity.

A moist, frothy tongue usually calls for biochemic Nat. Mur. as a medicine.

When the tongue is greyish-white at the base this points to the liver.

A greenish coating also suggests liver and/or bowel trouble.

A red tongue indicates inflammation such as gastritis. Also fever.

When the tongue is mapped there may be pancreatic trouble.

A red tip may point to acidity and rheumatism.

A white tongue almost always means that the liver is sluggish.

A yellow coating indicates acidity, and often a bad liver as well.

TONSILS

The tonsils are detoxicating organs, and were placed in the body for a purpose. When the body is toxic they enlarge to deal with the poisons, so why cut them out? That does not remove the cause. There are cases occasionally where the tonsils themselves have become so poisonous as to be a source of infection, and in such cases they may have to be removed. But, very few cases call for surgical interference; they can be corrected by sensible dieting (see **Diet**), breathing exercises, throat packs and medicine. Treatment may be administered as for **Auto-toxaemia**. Excellent homoeopathic remedies are as follows. For enlarged tonsils give five pills of Phytolacca 3. before meals, and four of Baryta Carb. 6. after meals, three times daily. Also three tablets of Kali Mur. 6x on rising and retiring. When the tonsils are septic give four pills of Phytolacca 3 before meals and four of Drosera 3 after meals three times daily; also Kali Mur 6x (three tablets) morning and night. If fever is present give Aconite 3 instead of the Drosera until the fever has subsided. When there is a Nat. Mur., type of tongue give three tablets of Nat. Mur 6x instead of the Kali Mur.

The throat may be sprayed twice daily with the mother tincture of Hydrastis (Golden Seal). See also under **Sore Throat**.

TOOTH-ACHE

The repeated suppression of pain in the teeth can be dangerous, as a bad tooth can be a focal point of infection, and poison the entire organism. Visit the dentist regularly, and have any bad teeth extracted.

Bathing the face and the back of the neck with very hot water will often bring relief from pain. Another method is to plug the cavity with a little cotton wool saturated with oil of Cloves; also rub the gums with the oil. Anti-spasmodic drops will sometimes take away the pain. Take a dose in hot water every half an hour. (See **Spasmodic Troubles**.) In some instances to plug the cavity with the drops acts better than Clove oil. Yet another way is to fill the cavity with equal parts of chloroform and homoeopathic Plantago mother tincture, and renew every ten minutes until the pain has gone. The gums may be gently massaged with the same tincture. Sometimes, four pills of Belladonna 3. every fifteen minutes for four to six doses, will relieve toothache. Or, try Ferr. Phos. 3x or 6x, or Mag. Phos. 6x (dissolve 10 tablets) in hot water in frequent sips. Note that when the pain is better for cold give Ferr. Phos.; if relieved by heat give Mag. Phos.

An old remedy used in the seventeen-hundreds was to burn brandy on a pewter plate, keep the opposite nostril stopped, and sniff up the hot brandy fumes frequently. Inhaling the fumes of volatile oil of Mustard is also claimed to be a cure, and in some cases the effect is immediate.

Do not forget that bad teeth point to errors in diet, and too many sweets. To help correct dental defects take two tablets of Calc. Phos. 3x before meals, and two of Calc. Fluor. 6x after meals. Also three tablets of Silica 6x or 8x on rising, and again on retiring. Keep this up for several weeks; only good can result.

Vegetable charcoal, used as a toothpowder, will keep the teeth clean and white, and disinfect the mouth far better than the much-advertised tooth pastes. Common salt is also good. Children like to use good quality sugar of milk (from chemists). This absorbs deposits and clears away tartar.

Before a tooth extraction take one dose of homoeopathic Hypericum 30 (five pills) and take another dose after the extraction. Also, add a small teaspoonful of homoeopathic Calendula mother tincture to half a glass of tepid water, sip occasionally and hold in the mouth for a minute or so; if still bleeding eject the residue; if not bleeding the Calendula may or may not be swallowed. Take another dose of Hypericum 30 on retiring.

TOXAEMIA (see AUTO-TOXAEMIA)

TYPES OF PEOPLE

A great deal has been written about types and constitutions, and much of the information is valuable to practitioners, but rather complicated for the average reader. However, it makes life easier for us all if we understand each other, and for our purpose we shall deal very briefly with the three basic types of individual. If we get a fair idea of these three types and how they react to circumstances and people, we shall be less likely to pass judgement on their actions. Also, if we understand to which type we belong to personally, we can get more out of living, and keep ourselves healthier and happier. The three types are the physical, the spiritual or emotional and the intellectual.

The physical type is 'of the earth earthy'. He or she is usually thick-set, of ruddy complexion and very fond of food. The head of the physically based is largest at its base: round the ears — a wide head. Of course, every individual has all three departments in his make-up; we are at the same time physical, spiritual and intellectual beings; it is the largest department in our make-up that determines our basic type; but each of the three types has his first and second inclinations. Thus, the physical type may be strongly inclined to spiritual matters, and the spiritual side becomes his first inclination. That leaves the intellectual side of the triangle his weakest inclination. Or, the inclinations may be the reverse. It is not wise to expect a strong physically based individual to act like an intellectual; or, a spiritual type to react to circumstances in the same manner as a physical type.

The physical type make excellent farmers, and if the spiritual inclinations are strong they make good preachers. The celebrated preacher, Spurgeon, was of this type. If the intellectual inclination is the strongest, then our physically based individual will do well in intellectual matters. A physically based person with a strong spiritual inclination would make a poor business man, but he would probably do well in business if his first inclination was intellectual. Do not expect a strong physical type who is intellectually inclined to understand a spiritual type. They do not speak the same language.

Of course, the ideal type is where the two inclinations are fairly well developed. This well balanced person is likely to be full of understanding, possessed of many abilities and be all things to all men. Indeed, it is not easy to 'base' the well-balanced individual.

Each type has a basic organ, and as long as his basic organ is healthy he can throw off all manner of ailments. Once his basic organ is affected he is a very sick person. The physically based type likes strong colours, is favourably affected by red, and his basic organ is his liver. Hence, to keep well he, or she, should avoid foods that put too much strain on the liver. When you meet the physical type try to understand how he thinks and acts, and do not blame him when he just cannot understand matters that are beyond his comprehension, or are not in line with his chief inclination.

The spiritual or emotionally based is usually a thin person, inclined to stoop and has a high, somewhat receding forehead. If his forehead is upright and square he is not spiritually based — he would be intellectually based, but have a very strong spiritual first inclination; in this case the physical would be the weakest inclination. The spiritual type takes to spiritual matters as a duck takes to water; he is found among the capable preachers, humanitarians, poets and artists. Of course that at which he excels will depend very largely on the strength of his first inclination. All shades of blue have a favourable effect on this type. His basic organs are the kidneys and generatives, and he will maintain a fair state of health for as long as these organs are functioning normally. This type requires plenty of fresh salads in his diet.

A very fine example of a spiritually based person was the late Pastor Russell, but both his inclinations were so strongly developed that he would have made a success in business, as a farmer, an actor, an engineer or in any form of occupation. The strongly based spiritual type with poor inclinations is a difficult person to understand, as he is not practical and wants to live in the heavens with his feet off the earth. When you contact this type, keep this in mind, and you will understand him better.

The intellectual type is usually well-built with a prominent, high forehead. But remember that his appearance is largely determined by the strength of his first inclination. If the physical side is poor he will not be so well built. This type make good investigators, teachers, scientists and actors. When their inclinations are strongly developed they are truly wonderful people. They take care of the affairs of mankind. On the other hand, when, for example, their spiritual inclination is the weakest they are most intolerant of spiritual matters and tend to make a god of their own intellect. Do not expect to be understood by such a person; but, with this knowledge, *you* can understand him. When this type is well-balanced they are the salt of the earth; when the spiritually is poor they may be most clever in their activities, but they can equally make expert criminals. The late William Gladstone was a good example of an intellectually based man with strongly developed inclinations. A very fine type indeed.

The basic organs of the intellectually based are the lungs,

and as long as the respiratory organs are healthy they can throw off other ailments. Once the lungs weaken they are very sick. It is this type that so easily become victims of T.B. They react favourably to yellow and brown, and require plenty of fresh fruit.

In marriage a knowledge of the type of partner is most helpful. It is wise to select a partner with a different base, but the first inclination of the proposed partner should be of the same base as yourself, or his or her first inclination the same as your first inclination. Thus, a physically based person should make a success of marriage to either an intellectually or spiritually based type, provided the partner has either a first physical inclination, or his or her first inclination is the same as that of your own. If you are physical with, say, a first inclination spiritual, your partner's first inclination should be either the same as your base (physical) or the same as your first inclination (spiritual). The children of such unions have a better chance for health and success in living. If the physically based selects a partner of the same base they may not get on well together; but if their first inclinations are the same they may do well. If the partner's first inclination is not the same as your base or your first inclination, but the same as your weakest inclination, then such a union is likely to be unhappy.

All three types can be excellent people, and one type cannot boast of his superiority in that he is, say, an intellectual. All types are good and necessary; all should strive to grow in mind, body and spirit and aim at being well-balanced individuals. It does not follow that a strongly spiritually based individual must be interested in theology; he may be an atheist. What one may be certain about is that whatever his views he will be very emotionally active either as an exponent of matters spiritual, ideological or political.

THE PHYSICAL BASE

Appearance of the true type: Thick-set. A strong body. The head is roundish and wide over the ears; not a very prominent forehead and not high in the crown of the head.

Basic organ: Liver.

Essential item in diet: Whole grain foods.

Favourite colour: Red.

Occupation: Farmer. Work calling for manual effort. Also, any profession or occupation with the first (strongest) inclination.

Inclinations: If the forehead is fairly pronounced and the top and back of the head is not so evident, then the first inclination is intellectual. If the forehead recedes and the crown of the head is fairly well in evidence, then the first inclination is spiritual.

THE SPIRITUAL BASE

Appearance of the true type: Slender build. Sometimes inclined to stoop. The forehead tends to recede slightly, or in a pronounced manner, and the head is narrower than that of the physical type. But, if the first inclination is physical, this type will display some width over the ears, and the body will be fairly well developed.

Basic organs: Kidneys. Also the generatives.

Essential item in diet: Green, leafy vegetables.

Favourite colour: Blue, and shades of blue.

Occupation: The ministry, or any pursuit associated with spiritual matters, the arts and humanitarian work. Selection depends largely on the first inclination.

Inclinations: If the forehead is fairly well developed and the individual has a narrowish head, the first inclination would be intellectual. If the forehead recedes and there is some obvious width over the region of the ears, then the first inclination would be physical.

THE INTELLECTUAL BASE

Appearance of the true type: This type has a good forehead; square, upright, or with a slight bulge. The body is usually well proportioned, although a strong spiritual first inclination may mean some slenderness. Usually the features are good and look intelligent.

Basic organs: The lungs.

Essential item in diet: Fresh fruits.

Favourite colour: Yellow, and shades of yellow.

Occupation: All intellectual and scientific pursuits. Also, acting and politics; the law.

Inclinations: If the physical features are the most pronounced, then that is the first inclination; if the spiritual signs are more obvious, then the first inclination is spiritual.

MARRIAGE AND PARTNERSHIPPS

Physical Base: Select an opposite base, but according to the strongest inclination. Thus, the partner should be intellectually or spiritually based, but have his or her first inclination physical, or the same as your own first inclination.

Spiritual Base: The partner should be physically or intellectually based, or his first inclination spiritual, or the same as your own.

Intellectual Base: Select a spiritual or physical base, with the first inclination intellectual, or the same first inclination as your own.

TYPHOID

It will require a trained diagnostician to detect typhoid, and it is important that the sufferer be placed under expert supervision. Herbal practitioners and homoeopaths can deal with typhoid very effectively, and without using dangerous drugs. Remedies which deal with this condition are Anacardium, Lachesis, Millifolium, Plumbum, Aesculus and several others which are selected according to the type of patient and symptoms exhibited. Rightly used, Anacardium is a wonderful remedy for typhoid.

Among the helpful herbal remedies are Echinacea, Bayberry, Pleurisy root and Ginger. Directions for home treatment are not given as we believe this should be entirely in the hands of the experienced practitioner.

ULCERS

Treat as for **Abscess**. See also **Auto-toxaemia, Potato, Poultices.**

UNICORN ROOT (TRUE)

In herbal medicine the root of this plant is employed as a tonic and digestive, and for weakness of the female generative organs. It will prove most helpful whether given in material doses or in homoeopathic form. Experience shows that for prolapse of the uterus, and when that organ is not in position, Unicorn Root (Aletris Farinosa) in the 30th. potency has few equals as a remedy. For prolapse and malposition of the uterus we recommend five pills of Aletris Farinosa 30. morning and night for three or four weeks. Or, take fifteen drops of the fluid extract in a little hot water before meals, three times daily. But we advocate this excellent remedy in the homoeopathic form.

URINE THERAPY

The idea of using one's urine medicinally is unpleasant, especially to the so-called civilised, refined(?) people. Let us remember that 'Nothing is good or bad but thinking makes it so'. Urine has been employed for remedial purposes during the whole of recorded history, and is being used today with the most satisfactory results. It is employed both internally and externally for a variety of ailments. Some practitioners give the sufferer's urine in potency, when it is not objectionable, as it has been so highly diluted. From the homoeopathic standpoint it fulfils the law of 'like cures like', for one's urine contains traces of the causes which produce disease; hence, by administering these toxic substances in homoeopathic form the disease is eliminated. However, the same law seems to operate when the urine is not diluted, probably owing to the fact that the active properties are present in very small quantities, and also because the urine is, by nature, not poisonous to its owner. Strictly speaking this is not homoeopathy, and the method is known as isopathy.

We know of a lady of advanced years who has the skin and appearance of a very young and healthy woman. She came forward after one of our lectures and gave the information privately to the speaker that her health and youthfulness were due to the fact that she took some of her own urine daily. The subject had been mentioned during the lecture. We know of one very bad case of rheumatoid arthritis, with an associated skin disease, cured by the sufferer's own urine. But, it is very difficult to get people to take this treatment in crude form. More will take their urine potentised, when they get similar good results. Just a few have been given their own urine in homoeopathic form without their knowledge, and have put down their cures to our 'wonderful remedies'.

In country districts it is not unusual for housewives to rub their hands with their own urine morning and night. This certainly keeps the hands free from hard skin, chaps and chilblains. We have seen farmers' wives with hands like those of a child, and they have confessed that the reason has been the use of urine. This was true years ago when we lived in the country; probably few do this today, as most women would be caught up by the advertisements for fancy creams and lotions. Urine, applied to cuts and sores, by means of bandages soaked therein, has speeded up healing and caused healthy flesh to replace abnormal tissue.

A wineglassful or more of morning urine taken three times daily before meals, has performed the seemingly impossible for cases of arthritis, rheumatism, skin disease of a stubborn character, chilblains and general debility; also for acid dyspepsia. For those who allow reason to rule over feelings this method could be tried, as it is positively harmless, and may be resorted to when other remedies fail. Those who cannot bring themselves to take neat urine can resort to a prepared potency of their early morning urine. Some homoeopathic chemists will undertake to make the 'medicine', although the process takes time and the sufferer must be prepared to pay the cost. The 6th. potency is recommended in liquid form. Dose: about five drops in a teaspoonful of water before meals, three times daily. Homoeopathically prepared in the 6th. potency, urine is tasteless. In fact the actual substance is no longer present; what remains is a powerful healing *force*. In some instances the 30th. potency would be more effective, but this would cost more to make. If the 30th. potency is employed the dose should be five drops in water morning and night. Treatment may be continued for as long as necessary.

UTERUS PROLAPSE

Prolapse of the uterus has been remedied by such medicines as Witch Hazel, (Hamamelis), Unicorn root (Aletris Farinosa), Murex, Lilium Tig., Agaricus and Fraxinus. (See under headings for the first two.) Should Witch Hazel or Unicorn fail, try the others, one at a time, in homoeopathic potency. The 30th. potency is advised. Take five pills of the selected remedy morning and night for three weeks. If better, but not normal, continue the remedy for a little longer.

Unicorn root (Aletris) will usually cure, either in homoeopathic or fluid extract form. We often give Aletris 30. on rising and Fraxinus 30. on retiring. Also two tablets of Calc. Fluor. 6x after meals. When falling of the womb, retroversion, etc., is accompanied by other troubles of the organ, it is sometimes necessary to give Murex 30. In such cases give a dose of Murex 30. before lunch, as well as the other selected remedy.

UVA-URSI

The leaves have been used for generations in the treatment of kidney and bladder disorders, catarrh of the urinary organs, stone, gravel, ulceration and leucorrhoea. There is ample evidence that Uva-Ursi acts as a tonic to the pancreas and colon. It seems to exert a favourable influence on mucous membranes everywhere, acting not only as a cleansing agent, but as a strengthening tonic.

Simmer an ounce of the leaves in one pint of water for ten minutes, in an iron or enamel pot. Strain. Dose: a tablespoonful to a wineglassful before every meal. This remedy is one of the best of which we know for the disorders mentioned. The fluid extract may be used, although it is not so effective as the infusion. Dose for the fluid extract is half to one small teaspoonful in hot water before meals.

VACCINATION

The bad effects of vaccination usually respond to homoeopathic Thuja 30. For infants dissolve two pills in a feed once daily for four days. Or, dissolve three pills of Thuja 3. in a feed once daily for ten days.

VALERIAN

At one time Valerian was the chief remedy employed by herbalists for almost all nervous complaints; and very good it is. It is ideal for all cases of nervous debility, hysteria, irritation and nerve pains. There are absolutely no harmful effects. Pronounced cases of neurasthenia have been cured by this simple remedy. Place an ounce of the herb in an iron or enamel pot. Pour on a good pint of boiling water, and simmer gently with the lid on for ten minutes. Strain. Take a wineglassful before every meal, and in cases of insomnia, an additional dose on retiring. The fluid extract, which is almost as good as the tea, is taken in half teaspoonful doses in hot water.

VARICOCELE

This is a condition of dilated veins in the spermatic cord. It usually affects the left testicle more than the right. In many instances the cause is due to masturbation in youth. The testicles should be bathed with a teaspoonful of distilled extract of Witch Hazel in a tumbler of cold water, twice daily. Internally, take five pills of Pulsatilla 30. on rising, and two tablets of Ferr. Phos. 6x after meals, three times daily. The condition is not regarded as serious and many men have varicocele for their adult lifetime, with no ill effects.

VARICOSE VEINS

Varicose veins are among the most difficult troubles to cure, and very often the best treatment fails. It has been noticed, however, that when, for reasons of illness, a sufferer has to stay in bed for a period of several weeks, the veins become normal. Unfortunately, they do not remain so for long. The rest in the horizontal position relieves the pressure in the veins which is present when one is in the upright position and gives the collapsed and weakened valves in the veins a chance to recover. When proper treatment is given under these conditions there is a good chance that the trouble may not return; or, at least, not so badly. Treatment when one has to be about every day is not so easy, but the following advice has produced some very good results in many cases.

When possible apply compresses of distilled extract of Witch Hazel to the veins. Such applications, even for a short period during the day, are helpful. The better plan is to wear them all night. Witch Hazel may also be taken internally: two or three drops in a wineglass of cold or tepid water every three hours for as long as is necessary.

Homoeopathic treatment has produced some very fine results. Take five pills of Secale 30. on rising, and five of Iodine 30. on retiring nightly. Also two tablets of Ferr. Phos. 6x before lunch and the evening meal, and two of Calc. Fluor. 6x after these two meals. Females who are fair and inclined to stoutness will usually derive more benefit if Pulsatilla 30. is taken in place of the Iodine. In cases of high blood pressure with varicose veins this condition should receive attention before treating the veins. Do not wear elastic hose. In bad cases a very wide crêpe bandage may be used; but never bind tightly.

Every night on going to bed stroke the veins upwards towards the heart for a few minutes with the dry hands, or with extract of Witch Hazel.

VERVAIN

An excellent remedy for spasmodic nervous conditions, and very useful in the early stages of fevers. Also useful for spasmodic coughs. Prepare a tea in the usual way: one ounce to a pint of water simmered gently for ten to fifteen minutes. Strain. To children, for coughs, colds and feverish conditions with nervous symptoms, give a dessertspoonful to a tablespoonful, according to age, three or four times daily. The dose for adults is a wineglassful three or four times daily. Larger doses may cause vomiting; but Vervain is harmless. For the young the medicine should be sweetened, or flavoured with Liquorice.

The dose for the fluid extract is ten to fifteen drops for children, and half a teaspoonful for adults, in hot water.

VINEGAR AND BROWN PAPER

For quinsy, sore throat and laryngitis steam the throat with the following. In a suitable bowl or large pot place a pint of common Vinegar and then pour on a quart of boiling water. Cover the head with a towel to confine the steam, and inhale. It is claimed that this simple method has saved many lives. A cold Vinegar compress applied to the forehead will often give relief in headaches and fevers.

Vinegar is not advisable as an item in the daily diet. Use pure Lemon juice instead. Certainly, anaemic people should never touch it. There is evidence that Vinegar has caused anaemia. That is why some cases of anaemia may be cured by giving acetic acid (Vinegar) in homoeopathic form. However, Vinegar may be taken occasionally as a medicine when the liver is upset and there is a deficiency of acid in the stomach.

In such cases Vinegar, one to three teaspoonsful after meals, will often prove helpful. But it does not cure the cause; it is for relief only.

Vinegar, massaged thoroughly into the spine, will act as a tonic to the entire system. A special strong Vinegar (acetic acid) for spinal and other external treatment; is very effective. Acetic Acid can be obtained from most chemists, and instructions are given with the bottle.

Fever cases experience considerable relief when sponged down with cold or tepid Vinegar. Brown Paper, soaked in Vinegar, well-prepared (preferably with Cayenne pepper) and applied to the chest, will be of service in bronchitis and other respiratory troubles. This makes a quickly-prepared poultice for application to any painful area, and is far better than many of the poultices that are difficult to prepare. Such an application is also excellent for toothache and neuralgia. A cup of vinegar added to the usual bath water has a fine tonic effect. See also **Apple Cider Vinegar.**

In cold weather, sheets of brown paper, placed between the sheets or blankets, will prove very effective for keeping in the warmth.

VIOLET

Fresh Violet leaves are wonderful blood cleansers, and also have considerable value as a remedy for coughs and respiratory disorders. The fresh leaves are far better than the dry, but the latter may be used when fresh leaves are not obtainable. The most serious disorders due to impure blood and a toxic condition of the system have been cured by drinking Violet tea. Owing to its cleansing action on the system, Violet tea is also excellent for producing a healthy complexion.

Pour a pint of boiling water over a handful of the fresh leaves, and allow to stand for twelve hours. After this time has elapsed take a large wineglassful before every meal. While using up one infusion another can be in course of preparation. The dried leaves may be used in the same manner. For sores and ulcers apply lint soaked in the same infusion, and allow to remain on for three hours, then renew. An application can remain on all night. Violet tea may be taken for as long as may be necessary.

VITAMINS

It is only in recent years that Vitamins have been discovered. First of all these accessory food factors were suspected to exist. Investigation followed and they were discovered. Others are being added to the list of those Vitamins already known. As the name suggests, Vitamins are vital, life-giving substances. They are present in natural foods in small but essential quantities. How did people manage before Vitamins were discovered? The truth is that if a diet is simple, and consists of a variety of natural, unadulterated, unspoilt foods there is no need to worry about Vitamins. The chief Vitamins, their sources and their main uses are as follows:

Vitamins A. and D. Foods rich in these Vitamins are stated in their order of importance, those richest in the Vitamins being mentioned first. Fish liver oils, fish liver, animal liver, fish roes, egg yolk, green vegetables, carrots, tomatoes, milk, fresh fruits, whole cereals. These two Vitamins enable the system to resist colds and disease and help to delay senility. Contribute to healthy bone growth.

Vitamin B. There are several B. Vitamins. Foods rich in B, given in their order of importance, are: dried Yeast, the germ of cereals, Yeast extracts, Bran, buckwheat, peanuts, dried peas, beans and lentils, wholemeal wheat, oats, rye, maize, whole rice, egg yolk, lean meats, fruit and vegetables. The B Vitamins give energy and ensure a healthy nervous system. Activate the liver.

Vitamin C. The foods rich in this Vitamin, in order of importance, are: Rose hips, Black currants, Parsley, sprouts, kale, Asparagus, cabbage, watercress, broccoli, orange juice, Cayenne pepper, loganberries, gooseberries, grapefruit, Rhubarb, Lemons, red currants, new potatoes, tomatoes, raspberries, beans, lettuce, swedes, milk, parsnips, carrots, beets, Dandelions, Onions, plums, bananas, apples.

Vitamin C helps to cleanse the system of impurities, brightens the mind and aids the body in resisting disease.

Vitamin E. Found in the germ of wheat and other cerals, whole wheat, green leaves and in some vegetable oils. Wheat germ oil is very rich in E. This Vitamin acts as a strengthening agent to the heart and generative organs.

Vitamin P. The chief natural sources are oranges, Lemons

(also the peel), grapes, plums, Prunes, Rose hips and grapefruit.

This vitamin tones the arterial system, especially the capillaries. Hence this food accessory retards old age and diseases due to deterioration of the arteries, and helps to prevent high blood pressure.

Within the scope of this book it is unecessary to mention the other known Vitamins; and, of course, much more could be said regarding the action of those quoted. What we wish to impress on the reader is that natural, properly grown foods will supply all the Vitamins necessary to maintain good health. In our opinion, synthetic vitamins are not so good as those obtained from natural sources.

VOICE (LOSS OF)

Homoeopathic Phytolacca 3. is helpful in many cases. Dissolve four or five pills on the tongue every two hours. Another good remedy when the vocal chords are much affected is Polygonium Aviculare. Take as for Phytolacca; or, take Polygonium one hour, and Phytolacca the next, alternately. See also under **Quinsy** and **Sore Throat**.

To help restore the voice moisten the thumb and dip it in powdered borax; press the borax to the back of the roof of the mouth and permit it to remain there for as long as possible without moving the tongue. When saliva fills the mouth allow it to trickle out into a receptacle. After a few minutes the remaining borax may be swallowed. Or, merely place a little borax on the tongue, and allow it to remain there for as long as possible before swallowing or ejecting. Do this every few minutes until speech returns. This method is sometimes used by professional singers and speakers.

Another method is to spray the throat occasionally with genuine tincture of Golden Seal (Hydrastis). Balm of Gilead (Populus Candicans) 1x is regarded as a fine remedy, it is also excellent for hard coughs. Dose: five pills three or four times daily.

VOMITING

The cause must be discovered and treated accordingly. A tea made with common Spearmint is an excellent remedy for simple vomiting; and plain Lemon juice is good when it is due to a sick stomach. Homoeopathic Ipecac. 3., five pills three or four times daily, is also a most effective remedy. If Ipecac. fails try Lobelia Inflata 3. in the same manner. Pulsatilla 3. suits those who vomit from eating fats, especially if they are blond and inclined to stoutness. For the vomiting of pregnancy see **Morning Sickness.**

WARTS

We suppose that thousands of warts have been 'charmed' away. When we were children the baker's wife over the road cured many cases, including a nasty crop on our middle finger. All she did was to moisten the wart with her saliva and mutter something. We do not profess to be able to supply the answer to the question as to how warts are cured in this manner. They undoubtedly are, and we must leave it at that. Maybe it is due to some form of thought transference from the charmer to the sufferer?

A certain type of person tends to produce warts. To the homoeopathic physician such are known as the sycotic type. A very popular remedy for long used by this school of medicine is Thuja. (See **Thuja.**)

Warts can be removed by painting them with strong acetic acid. When this is done a small hole should be cut in a piece of cardboard to fit over the wart and protect the surrounding skin, as the acid burns. Paint the wart two or three times daily, with the card in position. The fresh juice of the common Celandine may also be tried.

An old treatment was to scrape up a little dry pipe-clay and rub it on the wart three or four times daily. We have seen good results from this method.

The late Dr. Guyon Richards advocated homoeopathic Castoreum 30. for warts. Dose: five pills morning and night for two or three weeks. We have eliminated many bad warts with this remedy. Also, a horse which was covered with warts responded to Castoreum. We placed half a teaspoonful of Castoreum 30., in dilute spirit form, in the animal's mouth daily for six days. Thuja 30. had been tried previously with no result..

To apply a little Castor Oil to a wart two or three times daily had proved to be effective in many cases. Teatment has to be continued for some time.

Old country cures consisted of rubbing a wart daily with a cut radish or with the juice of Marigold Flowers, Celandine or Dandelion stems.

WETTING OF BED

This distressing condition may call for psychological treatment, as causes may be on the mental/emotional plane. Quite often it is the child's way of drawing attention and sympathy, although he may not be aware of the fact. There may also be physical causes. Bed-wetting (Enuresis) will sometimes yield to Mullein oil given in three to five drop doses before meals, three times daily. The recipe given under **Bladder Weakness** is also very good. When worms are the cause treat accordingly.

WHOOPING COUGH

There are several reliable herbal and homoeopathic remedies for this very distressing trouble, which can cause constitutional weakness for life if not eased up and eliminated. Even valvular heart weakness can be caused by whooping cough. Some herbalists regard Mouse-ear as a specific. Place an ounce in a jug; pour on one pint of boiling water; cover, and allow to stand for at least an hour. Then stir in four ounces of best Honey. For young children give two teaspoonsful every hour; or, immediately following a fit of coughing. Administer less frequently as the sufferer improves. For older children the dose may be increased up to a wineglassful.

Linseed is also a good remedy for whooping cough. Homoeopaths usually advise Sundew (Drosera) 3. Give two to five pills, according to age, three or four times daily. Another exceptionally good remedy is Ambra Gris. 30. For the acute stage give this remedy in doses of two to five pills every three hours, and less frequently as the condition improves. Ambra Gris. kills the virus.

A sniff of turpentine will often ward off an attack of coughing. It is a good thing to keep a saucer with a little turpentine in it somewhere in the sick room.

An old cure was to chop up a swede and cover with brown sugar. After standing for about twelve hours give the child a teaspoonful of the sugared juice immediately following every coughing attack. Note that the child should also take his meals after an attack, so that the food will not be vomited. Give plenty of Lemon or other pure fruit juices.

WILD CHERRY

An ingredient in many reliable herbal cough medicines. The dose for the fluid extract is half a teaspoonful in hot water, with Honey added, three or four times daily.

WILD INDIGO

This is the Baptisia of the homoeopaths. Two or three doses of Baptisia 200. have done much to remove the mental state of self-pity. Wild Indigo is a powerful antiseptic and is excellent for blood disorders and toxic conditions. It has proved to be most valuable in cases of fever and influenza. Has a special action on the bowels; and, according to Dr. Guyon Richards, is the best remedy for appendicitis. We, personally, have cleared up several cases of severe appendicitis by giving twenty drops of Baptisia C.M. potency every hour for six to eight hours. This approach to appendicitis by giving Baptisia in such high potency may amaze most homoeopaths, as it is so very unusual. But it certainly acts. The vomiting ceases and the pain disappears. Possibly, good results in such a condition would be obtained by giving the remedy in a much lower potency; but we have not tried it, so cannot say.

A word of warning. It is dangerous to experiment with a case of appendicitis, and the reader is advised to obtain the services of a homoeopath or herbalist. The condition can be wrongly diagnosed by the inexperienced, and sometimes by the professional healer. Hundreds are minus an appendix which should never have been removed, as the organ was quite healthy, and the pain nothing more than common tummy ache. One has to remember that if it is appendicitis, and treatment is delayed, the condition can turn into a very serious one. Hence the need for caution. One can always give Baptisia until a professional diagnosis has been made, and by that time Baptisia may have acted. If it is not appendicitis, then the Baptisia can only do good, as it is a grand remedy for all forms of bowel toxaemia.

WILD YAM

One of the best antispasmodics in the materia medica. Highly praised by the herbalists and the homoeopaths. Wild Yam (Dioscorea) acts on the stomach, liver, nerves and intestines. It also has some tonic value. Some practitioners believe it to be unequalled for bowel disorders accompanied by spasm and pain. It may be administered with absolute safety for any bowel complaint (with Baptisia for appendicitis).

The remedy may be used for indigestion when there is pain in the stomach, biliousness, nervous dyspepsia, colic and intestinal irritation. Half a small teaspoonful of the fluid extract in hot water, sweetened if desired, before or after meals, three times daily.

It is just as effective given homoeopathically, and in any of the lower potencies up to the 30th. For acute pain give four or five pills of Dioscorea 3. every hour until easier, and then three times daily. Chronic states may be treated by taking five pills of Dioscorea 30. on rising and on retiring for three or four weeks. The entire system benefits from this proven and reliable remedy.

WILLOW (BLACK)

This is given as a tonic to the generative organs, and has been found helpful for sexual neurasthenia, debility due to sexual excesses and lack of vitality. Has a direct action on the testicles and suprarenal glands. Dose: half a small teaspoonful of the fluid extract in hot water, three times daily. Or, five pills of Black Willow (Salix Nigra) 30. morning and night.

WINTERGREEN

Wintergreen is aromatic, astringent and stimulating. It is used chiefly as a remedy for rheumatism, and is one of the best known for this purpose. Simmer an ounce of the leaves in a pint of water for ten minutes only. Strain. The dose is a small wineglassful before or after every meal. The dose for the fluid extract is half a teaspoonful in hot water.

The oil may also be taken internally, when the dose is about five drops in a teaspoonful of brown sugar or Honey, two or three times daily. However, the oil is mainly employed as an external remedy for pains in the muscles and joints. It should be warmed and well massaged into the affected areas. Unfortunately, the genuine oil is difficult to obtain, and is expensive. The synthetic oil of Wintergreen is very effective, and enters into many rubbing oils for aches and pains. While it is not so good as the genuine oil it may be safely employed with hopes of success. The synthetic oil is known as methyl-salicylate, and is sold by all chemists.

WITCH HAZEL

This is a most valuable remedy for both internal and external use. It checks and helps to remove the cause of haemorrhages, tones the veins, arteries, ligaments, organs and skin. A decoction made from the bark or leaves forms an excellent injection for bleeding piles, and the same may also be applied externally to varicose veins on wide bandages. Apply the bandages well wetted with the decoction, but not tightly, and keep on all night. The wet bandages may be covered with dry towels.

Distilled extract of Witch Hazel may also be used as an application for vein troubles, and is very satisfactory. This extract is good for the skin of the face. Patted into the tissues it helps to remove wrinkles. Witch Hazel ointment is fine for piles, and it is often an ingredient in suppositories. Two or three drops of the extract in cold or tepid water before or after meals is a satisfactory medicine for prolapsed stomach and intestines, varicose veins, duodenal ulcers, haemorrhoids and internal haemorrhages. Applied externally it is also excellent for sores and wounds. Helpful in cases of nose-bleed, when a few drops may be placed in the palm of the hand and sniffed up the nose.

In homoeopathic form it is often more effective in the more chronic disorders of long standing. Take five pills of Hamamelis (Witch Hazel) 3. before every meal; or five pills of Hamamelis 30. on rising and retiring.

WOOD BETONY

A fine old remedy for nervous indigestion, skin diseases and rheumatism. Very good for nervous conditions which mainly affect the head. We found that people who always get a headache when their digestion is upset, respond very well to a tea of Wood Betony. Simmer an ounce in a pint of water, in an iron or enamel pot, for fifteen minutes, and then strain. Take a small wineglassful before meals, and again on retiring.

WORMS

Here is an ancient remedy which, so it is said, never fails to remove worms of all types, including tape-worm. Take about sixty fresh inner seeds of a pumpkin and a small teaspoonful of the fluid extract of Male Fern. Use less of the extract for young children. Well mix together in hot milk, and take the whole before retiring. Take a similar quantity first thing next morning, and no other breakfast food. An hour later give a dose of Epsom salts. Honey or Molasses may be added to make the gruel more palatable. Repeat, if necessary, in a few days.

The chief biochemic remedy for worms is Nat. Phos. 2x. Three tablets before every meal. However, we usually find that other remedies are also necessary. No doubt Nat. Phos. is helpful in removing the cause.

Another effective worm treatment consists of eating a small plateful of freshly shredded coconut. The coconut must be fresh. The milk from the nut should also be taken at the same time. This coconut is eaten for breakfast, and no other food taken. Have lunch as usual, but fast for the remainder of the day and have a similar coconut breakfast on rising. About two hours following this second breakfast take a dose of Epsom salts or castor oil, and the worms should come away. On rare occasions the breakfast, followed by a purgative, is necessary on the third day; but this is unusual. An injection into the bowel of a *tepid* infusion of Quassia is very effective in some cases.

Yet another method is to take two cloves of Garlic, boiled in a cupful of new milk and sweetened with Honey, on retiring. May be taken for several nights should this be necessary. Grated carrots sprinkled with Aniseed form a good worm remedy. Take for breakfast several days in succession. See also Wormseed.

It has been found that to anoint the anus with lard when there is any itching will give ease and prevent certain forms of worm eggs from hatching. An experienced investigator says that the female discharges its eggs around the anus. Lard applications two or three times daily destroy the larvae, and after a few days or weeks the sufferer is free from parasites. Dr. Woodvine of Boston confirms this discovery.

Some Homoeopaths recommend a dose of Sulphur 200 twice weekly for three weeks to deal with the constitutional condition irrespective of any local treatment.

Another medicine consists of adding Oil of Cade to the fluid extract of Tansy. Mix thoroughly by shaking the bottle. The dose is half a teaspoonful in a little water before or after meals, three times daily. To prepare the medicine add ten drops of Oil of Cade to eight ounces of Tansey extract. It is better not to exceed the dose, and this medicine should not be taken for more than two or three weeks. Give a slightly smaller dose to young children.

WORMSEED (CINA)

The botanic name for this is Cina, and it is one of the best worm remedies. Additionally, we find that, taken homoeopathically, it gives tone to the large bowel and has a soothing action on the abdomen as a whole. Has some value as a remedy for duodenal troubles. For worms it is used in material doses, or in homoeopathic form. We suggest three to five pills of Cina 3. before meals, three times daily. Cina ointment (from chemists and homoeopathic chemists) should be applied to the back passage at bedtime.

WORMWORD

An excellent remedy when there are spasms of the nervous system, trembling and hysteria. The action seems to be centered in the brain and spinal cord, and through these to all parts of the body. Wormwood should be considered as a remedy when there are marked nervous symptoms associated with congestive headaches, nervous indigestion, intestinal pain and spasms and reproductive troubles. We have found a cure for all these conditions in Wormwood when other treatments have failed; but always where there has been nervous disturbance. The remedy is also good for insomnia and vertigo. Lack of tone in the digestive organs will often respond to this fine remedy. We do not advise large doses. In the small doses, as advised, it is quite harmless. Infuse an ounce of the herb in a pint of boiling water, and allow to stand for half an hour. Dose: a tablespoonful before or after meals, and again on retiring for insomnia. Children less according to age. May be sweetened, or flavoured with Liquorice. Wormwood is also a cure for worms; hence its name.

Cases where the infusion failed to act have responded to Wormwood (Absinthium) 30. Five pills morning and night.

WOUNDS

First cleanse all wounds, and then apply cold water compresses. Or, use Marigold or Witch Hazel. Information is given under the headings. To stop bleeding apply a cold-water pad directly over the wound and bind fairly tightly. Keep the patient still and warm. If available give occasional doses of Arnica 3., Calendula 3. or Hypericum 3.

X-RAYS

The discovery of X-rays enabled phsyicians and surgeons to diagnose conditions which formerly could only be thought possible: duodenal ulcers, enlarged organs, prolapsed organs, growths, etc. Unfortunately these rays are dangerous to healthy tissue, and a series of X-ray photographs, or treatments, can result in damage. When used for healing the rays can destroy malignant growths, but in many instances the healthy tissues are also burnt, and this can cause the development of the same trouble in some other part of the body. (See also **Radiation**).

X-rays do not always disclose abnormal disease conditions. Owing to the locality of the trouble and the state of the tissues, a very obvious condition is occasionally not disclosed.

YARROW

A famous old herbalist, so it is said, used Yarrow for all sorts of complaints. His usual advice for colds, fevers, general upset, stomach and abdominal pains and many other conditions was to take a strong tea of Yarrow, piping hot, and get to bed with a hot brick to the feet. 'You will be all right tomorrow morning', he would say. The Yarrow tea usually acted. Why? Because Yarrow is one of the best of natural medicines for detoxicating the system, thus removing the causes of colds, aches and fevers. Yarrow stimulates the circulation, opens the pores of the skin and gives strength to the entire organism. There is plenty of evidence to prove that Yarrow has saved many lives; and it never has any harmful effect. Many practitioners add Elder blossom or Peppermint to the brew; and herbal Composition Powder also increases the curative value. An ounce of Yarrow simmered gently in one pint of water for about fifteen minutes is the usual way of preparing the medicine. Add a small teaspoonful of Composition Powder if you wish, and sweeten with honey to taste. Take a wineglassful, hot, every two hours, and a double dose at night. Always keep warm and never go out when taking hot Yarrow tea. It causes sweating, and the body easily takes a chill in such circumstances. See also the information given under Colds.

YEAST

Yeast is a Vitamin B food, and is of much value in disorders associated with a deficiency of this food accessory. Brewer's Yeast is better than that used by bakers. Plain Yeast tablets, obtainable from all chemists, are good for nervous indigestion, exhaustion and nervous troubles. But be sure to get the plain Yeast and not tablets containing crude minerals and suppressive drugs. Excellent Yeast foods which can be used as beverages or spreads are available in Health Food Stores and grocery shops.

YELLOW DOCK

Has a slightly laxative and tonic action, but is chiefly alterative when used in material doses. It is undoubtedly a fine blood cleanser, and has done much good in cases of acidity, rheumatism, skin diseases and toxaemia. For some reason most herbal works of reference have nothing to say concerning Yellow Dock as a remedy for coughs and lung congestion; yet, it is one of the best of cough medicines and a builder of the respiratory organs. We find that for chest and lung complaints it acts better in homoeopathic potency. Take five pills of Rumex Crispus (Yellow Dock) 3. every two hours for lung troubles; or, for chronic conditions, five pills morning and night of Rumex 30. Sometimes the 30th. potency will act better than the 3rd. in acute conditions; but if this is the right remedy it will act in almost any potency. For blood and skin disorders, and for rheumatism, the fluid extract may be used: half a teaspoonful in hot water before every meal.

YERBA SANTA

This is grown in California, and is one of the best medicines for bronchitis, asthma and lung troubles that comes from that part of the world. For any kind of respiratory trouble the dose is half a teaspoonful of the fluid extract in hot water before meals. It is pleasant to take. Give young children smaller doses. Combined with Grindelia it forms a most excellent medicine for asthma.

ZONE THERAPY

Dr. Fitzgerald, a physician with a considerable reputation, discovered that deep massage and pressure on certain zones of the body restored organic functional activity in all regions situated in the zones treated. Treatment was, and still is, applied mainly to the feet. The points of pressure are also located in the hands. Indeed, in some respects Zone Therapy is somewhat similar to the treatment of the meridians in Chinese Acupuncture. There are, however, marked differences in the two systems.

Briefly, the body is divided into ten zones, one of these zones being traced from each finger and corresponding toe and passing through the various organs located therein. Thus the zone from the little finger and small toe passes up and down the outside of the body, affecting the shoulder, ear, hip and the skin on that side of the anatomy. The zone from the thumb and the great toe, passes through the stomach, bladder, etc. Zones from the third and fourth right fingers and toes pass through the liver and right kidney; those from the left through the left kidney and heart, spleen, etc. Pressure, or deep massage, on certain points in these longitudinal zones affect all organs in those zones by some kind of reflex action. Zone Therapy is, in fact, a method of treating disease and malfunctioning organs by reflex action.

Many years of experience by competent healers have proved beyond all question of doubt that these points of healing exist, and the results of proper treatment are surprisingly good. As the method is harmless and only good results, we decided to give some information on the subject for use in the home. If the reader has a sick liver he is certain to find a small area of great tenderness to deep pressure on the right foot a little way below the third and fourth toes. Press with the thumb until the tender spot is found, and then press hard. Also, give deep, circular movements with the thumb — light massage is useless. Sometimes the pain is rather severe, and this shows the need for treatment. Continue to press and move the tissues over the bones with deep, small circular movements until the pain is much easier, or has gone. By that time the sick liver will have received a 'tonic treatment'. Of course, in most cases, treatment should be given daily, or two or three times weekly, to normalize an organ, or to eliminate a disorder. It is wise to get another person to apply the pressure and massage, so that the sufferer can relax as much as possible while under treatment, which should continue for several minutes, with pauses if necessary. Self-treatment is possible of course. A hot foot bath before a treatment relaxes the tissues and speeds up effects.

A painful spot a little way below the third and fourth toes on the left foot indicates that all is not well with the heart, and treatment should be given accordingly. Painful spots below the waist of the foot towards the heel (in both feet) indicate intestinal congestion or disorders. Naturally, the area corresponding to the appendix is on the sole of the right foot, about two inches from the back of the heel and half an inch inwards from the outer side of the foot. Keep pressing and you are bound to find the right spot for treatment. Appendicitis has been cured by applying treatment to this locality.

The thyroid gland is treated by applying deep massage or pressure to the ball of the feet below the great toe of each foot. The brain and pituitary gland are stimulated by treating the balls of the great toes themselves. Naturally, the gall bladder is near and slightly below the liver area, and more to the centre of the foot. The stomach area is located in both feet below the thyroid gland areas. People with stomach trouble are very tender here. Press about with the thumb until the tender spot is discovered and then get to work. The pancreas area is more to the centre of the foot, below the stomach area and partly on both feet. The spleen is about half an inch inwards from the outside of the left foot and slightly below the area corresponding to the pancreas. The spine area is along the length of the inside of the feet from the outer sides of the great toes to the heels. Press inwards to contact the bones and joints of the feet in this area, and any painful spots point to some spinal congestion or subluxation. Find the painful areas and treat them, and your spine will benefit as well as the entire nervous system. Trouble in the throat is treated at the waist of the great toe; either or both according to the side affected. The lungs and bronchial tubes are treated by applying massage and deep pressure across the central sections of the feet immediately below the middle toes. Eyes and ears receive benefit from treatment applied to the waists of the three middle toes, and also the waists of the little toes in some cases. For such conditions the area immediately below the waists of these toes should also be treated.

Prostate gland, uterus trouble and rectal disorders are treated from the back of the heels upwards to above the ankles. Apply deep massage and pressure on both sides of the Achilles tendons, and the surrounding tissues.

All the zones are said to be present in the nose and rectum. This may explain the good results obtained from dilation of the rectum. Nature provides for this with every bowel evacuation when the stool is normal. Some years ago a certain man, whose name escapes memory, did very good work by inserting instruments into the nose to cause pressure, thereby stimulating all the zones.

The following diagrams will serve as a guide to home treatment with Zone Therapy. Note that any organ or locality through which a zone passes may be treated from *any* painful point on that zone. The special points of treatment indicated have a more positive action on the organs mentioned. When treating any point on a zone the locality selected will, therefore, have a special effect on the organ indicated, and at the same time favourably influence all other organs in that zone. When treating organs, or anatomical parts that are in pairs — lungs, kidneys, shoulders — it is advisable to treat the corresponding areas in both feet, even when one organ or side of the body only is affected. This also applies to single organs that have corresponding areas in both feet, such as the stomach and thyroid gland.

Some practitioners use their thumb nails to exert deep pressure on very small areas. A little practice will enable you to decide whether to employ the thumb, thumb nail or a finger over any area. Always apply the pressure, or deep massage, where it hurts most.

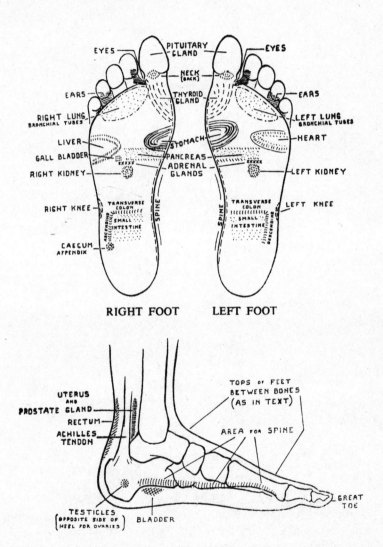

THE ZONES

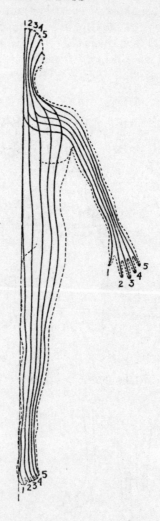

GENERAL INFORMATION

When fatigued, or feeling 'nervy', use an ordinary hair comb and stroke the palms of the hands with this, using gentle pressure, from the finger tips to the wrists (upwards) for a minute or two. Nervy people say this is most soothing. Similar treatment to the soles of the feet produces the same effect, but many are too ticklish for this form of foot treatment.

Although almost all practitioners of Zone Therapy treat the soles and sides of the feet, the zones may also be reached from the top of the feet. Trace, with deep pressure, up between the bones of the feet towards the ankles, and when a tender spot is found treat it thoroughly. The areas to be treated will be immediately above the corresponding areas on the sole of the foot. Occasionally, treatment of the top of the feet is more effective. If the area is very tender, then that is the area to receive attention no matter where it is located. Even if you are uncertain as to what any painful spot means, or what organ it represents, such a painful area indicates that something is wrong, and only good can result from treating that locality.

All painful places should receive a series of treatments until pain is no longer in evidence. After the first treatment, or treatments, each place may feel sore; but attention must continue until the pain has gone. We have helped all sorts of painful and congested conditions by this simple method, which can be done harmlessly at home by any moderately intelligent person. No matter what other treatment is given Zone Therapy can be employed as well. We recall stopping a case of severe hiccough that had gone on for many hours by pressing and giving deep massage on the centres of the soles of the feet for a few minutes. This is the solar plexus area, and treatment here helps in all nervous and spasmodic conditions.

OTHER METHODS

Most people know that a good way of helping an eye that has been irritated, or that has a particle of dust in it, is to rub the *other* eye. This acts reflexly on the affected eye and causes tears to flow, which swill out the obstruction. The treatment of opposite parts of the body can be applied for many conditions. For example: the shoulder corresponds to the hip; and one finds that if the right hip is painful there are tender places in the right shoulder when pressure is applied. Hence, a good way to help a painful right or left hip is to treat the right or left shoulder with deep massage and pressure on all painful spots.

There are also correspondencies between the shoulders and the joints of the small toes where they join the foot, and the little fingers where they join the hands. Manipulation of these joints and local tissues will, therefore, help any pain in the corresponding shoulders. Instead of manipulation, fomentations may be applied to the corresponding areas for several minutes. Use the water as hot as possible without scalding. We recall a case of neuritis in the right shoulder receiving speedy relief, and finally a cure, by the sufferer constantly dipping his right hand and wrist in very hot water. These simple things are well worth knowing, and can save an awful lot of suffering. Do not take notice of the clever people who dismiss these methods as being of no importance. What matters is relief from pain, and curing the conditions in a natural manner without poisoning the system with drugs.

A weak heart may be toned up, and pain in that organ relieved by working along between the ribs from the sternum (chest bone) towards the sides of the chest. Press deeply, and when a painful spot is discovered press and rub hard until the tenderness disappears. Several treatments may be required. The same applies to tender spots on the chest bone itself, and treatment of these places can help the body generally. A coughing spasm can be relieved by pressing on the top of the chest bone in the little hollow of the neck.

A case of severe toothache failed to respond to oil of Cloves and local hot fomentations on the painful side. The fomentations were then applied to the opposite side where no pain existed. Within a few minutes pain had gone on the affected side!. There is no doubt that hot foot baths affect the head (the opposite pole of the body), and not only help to equalize the circulation, but relieve congestion in the head, effects of high blood pressure, head colds, congestion in the ears, pains in the head and even help in some cases of mental dullness. On the other hand, vigorous massage of the scalp tends to benefit every part of the body. This stands to reason, as anything that stimulates circulation in the brain must have a good reflex action on the body, which is the physical expression of the individual — in a sense, the body is a product of the individual's total thinking. Hence, by improving brain function through better brain circulation the entire system benefits.

Strictly speaking, these methods of treatment by stimulating opposite parts of the body do not come under the heading of Zone Therapy; that system deals with reflex action along the zones only.

All the methods actually come under the heading of Reflex Therapy, or Reactopathy — a term we have personally applied to this system. This latter term implies that we are seeking to relieve or eliminate diseased conditions, and stimulate sluggish organs, by producing *reactions* through the treatment of other anatomical parts.

Of course, the affected organ itself should receive what attention is necessary, and the system under discussion must be regarded as an additional method of treatment. On occasions it proves to be all that is required when used intelligently.

While dealing with the feet it is interesting to note that hot bran poultices applied to those members for an hour or so, or at night to remain on until the morning, will do a great deal to build up the vitality of weakly people and ailing children. The entire organism benefits. For colds, sore throats, loss of voice and respiratory trouble a cold poultice of crushed garlic is excellent, although the aroma may annoy some people. This was John Wesley's remedy for such troubles.

THE COMMON AND BOTANICAL NAMES
OF HERBS MENTIONED IN THIS BOOK

Acacia (*Acacia Arabica*)
Agrimony (*Agrimonia Eupatoria*)
Angelica (*Angelica Archangelica*)
Arnica (*Arnica Montana*)
Arrowroot (*Maranta Arundinacea*)
Asafoetida (*Ferula Foetida*)
Balm (*Melissa Officinalis*)
Balm of Gilead (*Populus Candicans*)
Barberry (*Berberis Vulgaris*)
Bayberry (*Myrica Cerifera*)
Black Willow (*Salix Nigra*)
Bladderwrack (*Fucus Vesicolosus*)
Blue Flag (*Iris Versicolor*)
Boneset (*Eupatorium Perfoliatum*)
Broom (*Cytisus Scoparius*)
Bryonia (*Bryonia Alba*)
Buchu (*Barosma Betulina*)
Burdock *Arctium Lappa*)
Cade Oil *(Oleum Cadinum)*
Cajaput (*Melaleuca Leucadendron*)
Camphor (*Cinnamomum Camphora*)
Caraway (*Carum Carvi*)
Cardamoms
   (*Elettaria Cardamomum*)
Castor Oil (*Ricinus Communis*)
Catnep (*Nepeta Cataria*)
Cayenne (*Capsicum Minimum*)
Celandine (*Chelidonium Majus*)
Centaury (*Erythraea Centaurium*)
Chamomile (*Anthemis Nobilis*)
Chestnut (*Castanea Vesca*)
Chickweed (*Stellaria Media*)
Cinnamon
   (*Cinnamomum Zeylanicum*)
Cloves (*Eugenia Caryophyllata*)
Clubmoss (*Lycopodium Clavatum*)

Cohosh (Black)
   (*Cimicifuga Racemosa*)
Cohosh (Blue)
   (*Caulophyllum Thalictroides*)
Colchicum (*Colchicum Autumnale*)
Coltsfoot (*Tussilago Farfara*)
Comfrey (*Symphytum Officinale*)
Damiana (*Turnera Aphrodisiaca*)
Dandelion (*Taraxacum Officinale*)
Echinacea (*Echinacea Angustifolia*)
Elder Flowers (*Sambucus Nigra*)
Elecampane (*Inula Helenium*)
Eryngo (*Eryngium Campestre*)
Eucalyptus (*Eucalyptus Globulus*)
Euphorbium
   (*Euphorbium Resinifera*)
Evening Primrose
   (*Oenothera Biennis*)
Eyebright (*Euphrasia Officinalis*)
Gelsemium (*Gelsemium Nitidum*)
Gentian (*Gentiana Lutea*)
Ginger (*Zingiber Officinale*)
Ginseng (*Panax Quinquefolium*)
Golden Rod (*Solidago Virgaurea*)
Golden Seal (*Hydrastis Canadensis*)
Grindelia (*Grindelia Camporum*)
Guaiacum (*Guaiacum Officinale*)
Hawthorn (*Crataegus Oxycantha*)
Hellebore (*Helleborus Nigra*)
Helonias (*Helonias Dioica*)
Hemlock (*Conium Maculatum*)
Henbane (*Hyoscyamus Niger*)
Hops (*Humulus Lupulus*)
Horehound (*Marrubium Vulgare*)
Horse Chestnut
   (*Aesculus Hippocastenum*)

Horsetail (*Equisetum Arvense*)
Hydrocotyle (*Hydrocotyle Asiatica*)
Hyssop (*Hyssopus Officinalis*)
Ignatia (*Strychnos Ignatii*)
Ipecacuanha
　(*Psychotria Ipecacuanha*)
Irish Moss (*Chondrus Crispus*)
Jaborandi (*Pilocarpus Jaborandi*)
Kola (*Cola Vera*)
Labrador Tea (*Ledum Latifolium*)
Ladies' Slipper
　(*Cypripedium Pubescens*)
Lavender (*Lavandula Vera*)
Lily-of-the-Valley
　(*Convallaria Majalis*)
Lime Flowers (*Tilia Europeaea*)
Linseed (*Linum Usitatissimum*)
Liquorice (*Glycyrrhiza Glabra*)
Lobelia (*Lobelia Inflata*)
Lungwort (*Sticta Pulmonaria*)
Male Fern (*Dryopteris Filix-Mas*)
Mandrake (*Podophyllum Peltatum*)
Marigold (*Calendula Officinalis*)
Marjoram (*Origanum Vulgare*)
Marshmallow (*Althaea Officinalis*)
Meadowsweet (*Spiraea Ulmaria*)
Melilotus (*Melilotus Officinalis*)
Mistletoe (*Viscum Album*)
Motherwort (*Leonorus Cardiaca*)
Mountain Ash (*Pyrus Aucuparia*)
Mountain Flax
　(*Linum Catharticum*)
Mountain Laurel (*Kalmia Latifolia*)
Mousear (*Hieracium Pilosella*)
Mullein (*Verbascum Thapsus*)
Musk (*Moschus*)
Mustard (*Brassica Alba*, or
　Sinapis)
Myrrh (*Commiphora Myrrha*)
Nettle
　(*Urtica Dioica*) (*Urtica Urens*)
Night-Blooming Cereus
　(*Cactus Grandiflorus*)
Nutmeg (*Myristica Fragrans*)
Nux Vomica
　(*Strychnos Nux Vomica*)
Oak (*Quercus Robur*)
Oats (*Avena Sativa*)
Onion (*Allium Cepa*)

Orris (*Iris Florentina*)
Parsley Piert (*Alchemilla Arvensis*)
Passion Flower
　(*Passiflora Incarnata*)
Peach (*Prunus Persica*)
Pellitory-of-Wall
　(*Passiflora Incarnata*)
Pennyroyal (*Mentha Pulegium*)
Peony (*Paeonia Officinalis*)
Peppermint (*Mentha Piperita*)
Periwinkle (*Vinca Major*)
Peruvian Bark (*Cinchona Calisaya*)
Pilewort (*Ranunculus Ficaria*)
Pine (*Pinus Sylvestris*)
Pink Root (*Spigelia Marilandica*)
Pinus Bark (*Tsuga Canadensis*)
Plantain (*Plantago Major*)
Pleurisy Root (*Asclepias Tuberosa*)
Poison Oak (*Rhus Toxicodendron*)
Poke Root (*Phytolacca Decandra*)
Pomegranate (*Punica Granatum*)
Poplar (White)
　(*Populus Tremuloides*)
Poppy (*Papaver Somniferum*)
Prickly Ash
　(*Xanthoxylum Americanum*)
Primrose (*Primula Vulgaris*)
Psyllum (*Plantago Ovata*)
Puff Ball (*Lycoperdon Bovista*)
Pulsatilla (*Anemone Pulsatilla*)
Quassia (*Picraena Excelsa*)
Raspberry (*Rubus Idaeus*)
Red Clover (*Trifolium Pratense*)
Red Root (*Ceanothus Americanus*)
Red Sage (*Salvia Officinalis*)
Rhubarb (*Rheum Palmatum*)
Rosemary (*Rosmarinus Officinalis*)
Rue (*Ruta Graveolens*)
Sabadilla
　(*Schoenocaulon Officinale*)
Saffron (*Crocus Sativus*)
Sandalwood (*Santalum Album*)
Sarsaparilla (*Smilax Ornata*)
Sassafras (*Sassafras Officinale*)
Saw Palmetto (*Sereona Serrulata*)
Scullcap (*Scutellaria Laterifolia*)
Senna (*Cassia Acutifolia*)
Skunk Cabbage
　(*Symplocarpus Feotidus*)

Slippery Elm (*Ulmus Fulva*)
Southernwood
  (*Artemisia Abrotanum*)
Spearmint (*Mentha Viridis*)
Sponge (*Spongia Toasta*)
Squill (*Urginea Scilla*)
St. John's Wort
  (*Hypericum Perforatum*)
Stavesacre
  (*Delphinium Staphisagria*)
Stone Root
  (*Collinsonia Canadensis*)
Sumbul (*Ferula Sumbul*)
Sundew (*Drosera Rotundifolia*)
Sweet Vernal Grass (*Anthoxantum*)
Tansy (*Tanacetum Vulgare*)
Thuja (*Thuja Occidentalis*)
Thyme (*Thymus Vulgaris*)
Tolu Balsam
  (*Myroxylon Toluifera*)
Unicorn Root (*Aletris Farinosa*)

Uva-Ursi
  (*Arctostaphylos Uva-Ursi*)
Valerian (*Valeriana Officinalis*)
Vervain (*Verbena Officinalis*)
Violet (*Viola Odorata*)
Wild Cherry (*Prunus Serotina*)
Wild Indigo (*Baptisia Tinctoria*)
Wild Yam (*Dioscorea Villosa*)
Willow (Black) (*Salix Nigra*)
Wintergreen
  (*Gaultheria Procumbens*)
Witch Hazel
  (*Hamamelis Virginiana*)
Wood Betony (*Stachys Betonica*)
Wormseed (*Artemisia Cina*)
Wormwood (*Artemisia Absinthium*)
Yarrow (*Achillea Millifolium*)
Yellow Dock (*Rumex Crispus*)
Yerba Santa
  (*Eriodictyon Glutinosum*)

Where remedies in homoeopathic form have been stated in the text, and not their use as *material* medicines, they have not been included in this list, as the homoeopathic names *are* the botanic. Also, it has not been necessary to give the botanic names of all green vegetables that have been mentioned.